AF877841

It's easy to get lost in the cancer world

Let NCCN Guidelines for Patients® be your guide

- Step-by-step guides to the cancer care options likely to have the best results
- Based on treatment guidelines used by health care providers worldwide
- Designed to help you discuss cancer treatment with your doctors

National Comprehensive Cancer Network®

NCCN Guidelines for Patients® are developed by the National Comprehensive Cancer Network® (NCCN®)

NCCN

- An alliance of leading cancer centers across the United States devoted to patient care, research, and education

Cancer centers that are part of NCCN: NCCN.org/cancercenters

NCCN Clinical Practice Guidelines in Oncology (NCCN Guidelines®)

- Developed by doctors from NCCN cancer centers using the latest research and years of experience
- For providers of cancer care all over the world
- Expert recommendations for cancer screening, diagnosis, and treatment

Free online at NCCN.org/guidelines

NCCN Guidelines for Patients

- Present information from the NCCN Guidelines in an easy-to-learn format
- For people with cancer and those who support them
- Explain the cancer care options likely to have the best results

Free online at NCCN.org/patientguidelines

NATIONAL COMPREHENSIVE CANCER NETWORK
NCCN FOUNDATION
Guiding Treatment. Changing Lives.

and supported by funding from NCCN Foundation®

These NCCN Guidelines for Patients are based on the NCCN Guidelines® for Acute Lymphoblastic Leukemia (Version 1.2021, April 6, 2021).

NCCN Foundation seeks to support the millions of patients and their families affected by a cancer diagnosis by funding and distributing NCCN Guidelines for Patients. NCCN Foundation is also committed to advancing cancer treatment by funding the nation's promising doctors at the center of innovation in cancer research. For more details and the full library of patient and caregiver resources, visit NCCN.org/patients.

National Comprehensive Cancer Network (NCCN) / NCCN Foundation
3025 Chemical Road, Suite 100
Plymouth Meeting, PA 19462
215.690.0300

Endorsed by

Be The Match

Our Patient Support Center provides confidential, one-on-one support, counseling and educational resources. Our team is here if you want to learn about treatment options, ask questions, access financial grants, or talk with others. All of our programs and resources are free. Call 1 888-999-6743 or email: patientinfo@nmdp.org. bethematch.org/one-on-one

Stupid Cancer

Stupid Cancer helps to empower everyone affected by adolescent and young adult cancer by ending isolation and building community. We proudly support the NCCN Foundation's Mission to improve the care of patients with cancer. www.stupidcancer.org

The Leukemia & Lymphoma Society

The Leukemia & Lymphoma Society (LLS) is dedicated to developing better outcomes for blood cancer patients and their families through research, education, support and advocacy and is happy to have this comprehensive resource available to patients.lls.org/informationspecialists

To make a gift or learn more, please visit NCCNFoundation.org/donate or e-mail PatientGuidelines@nccn.org.

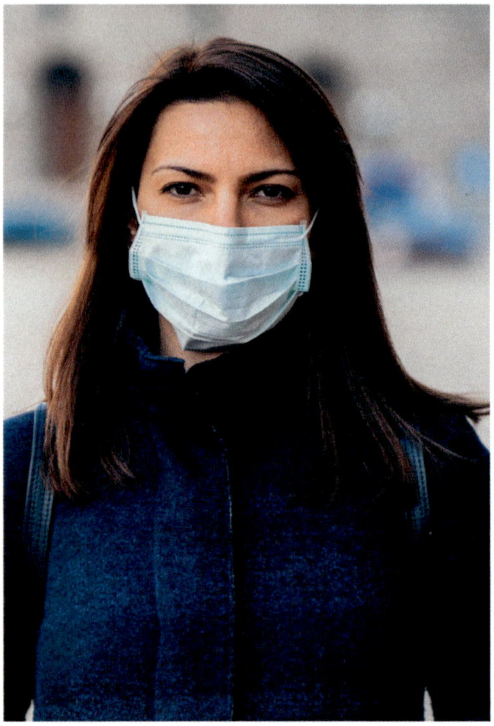
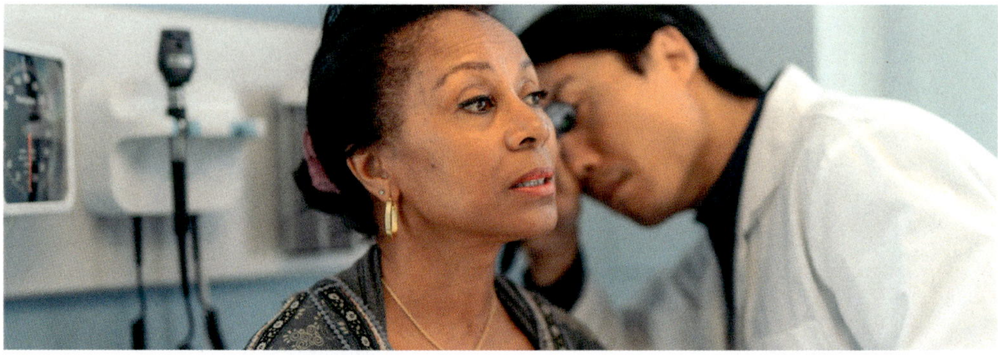
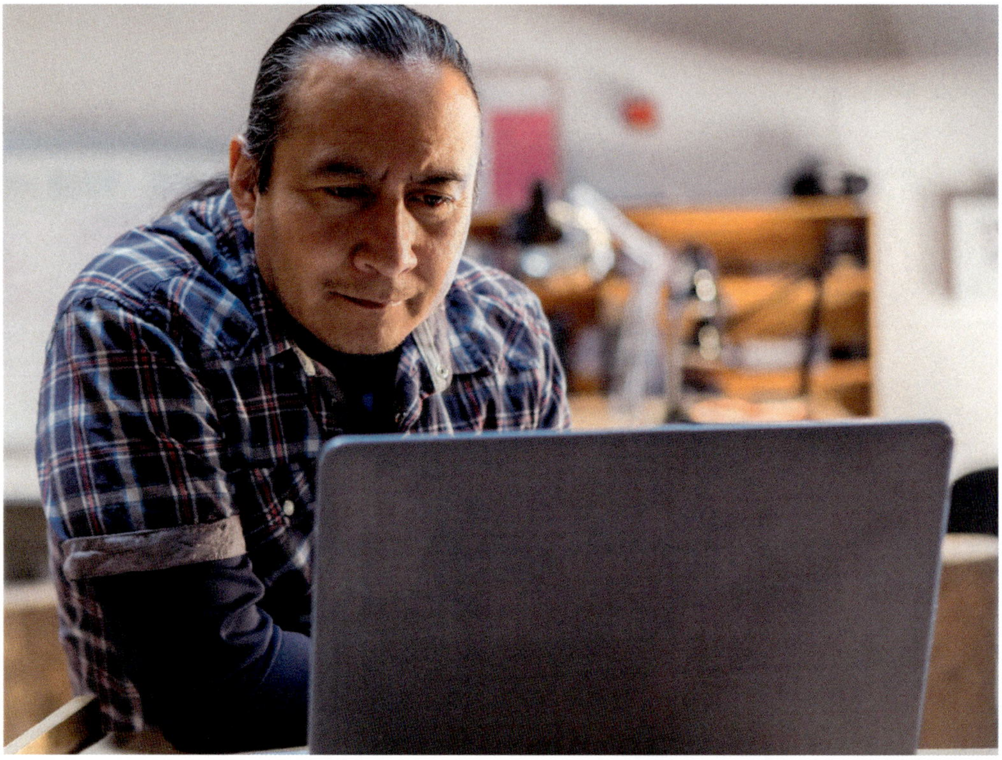
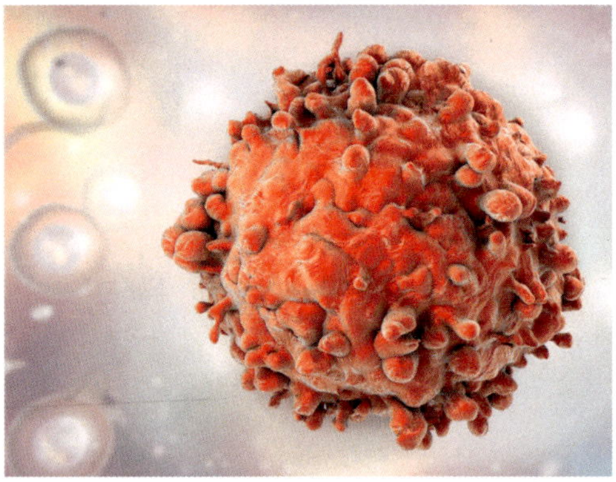
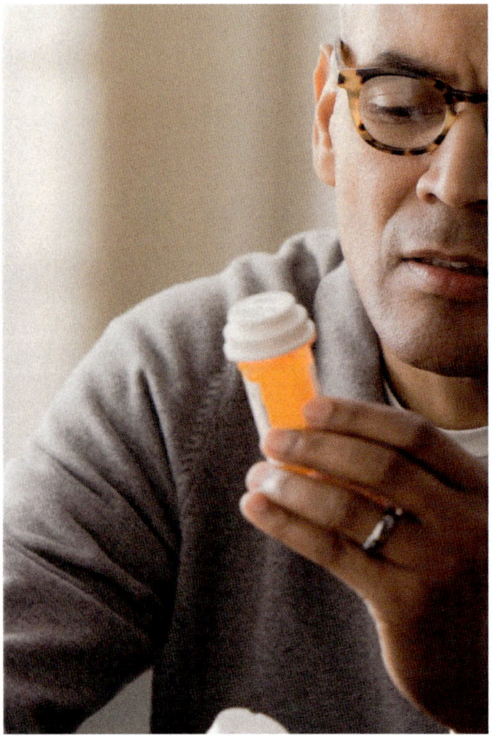
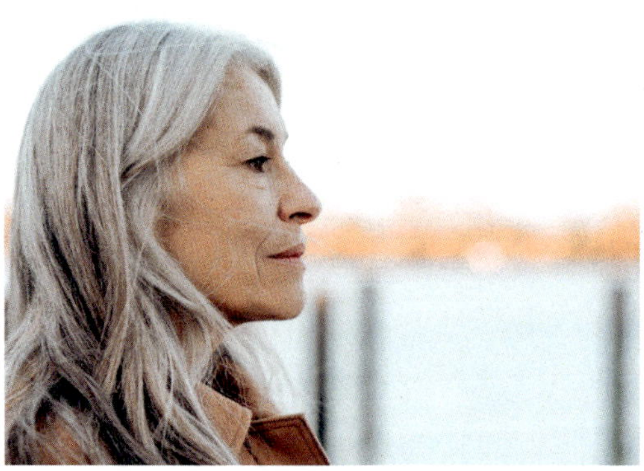
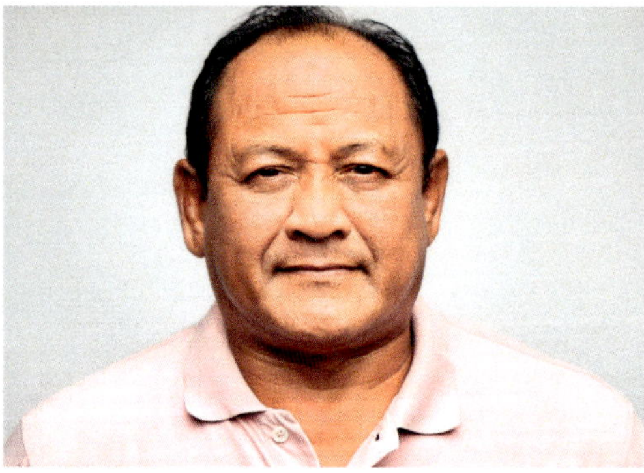
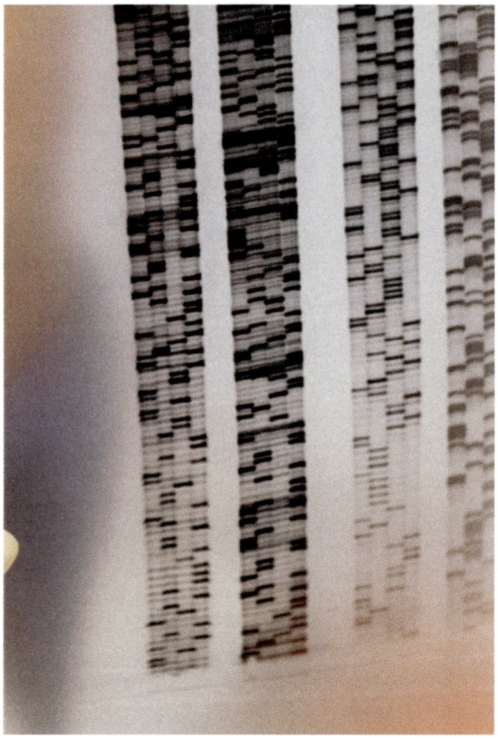

Contents

1
ALL basics

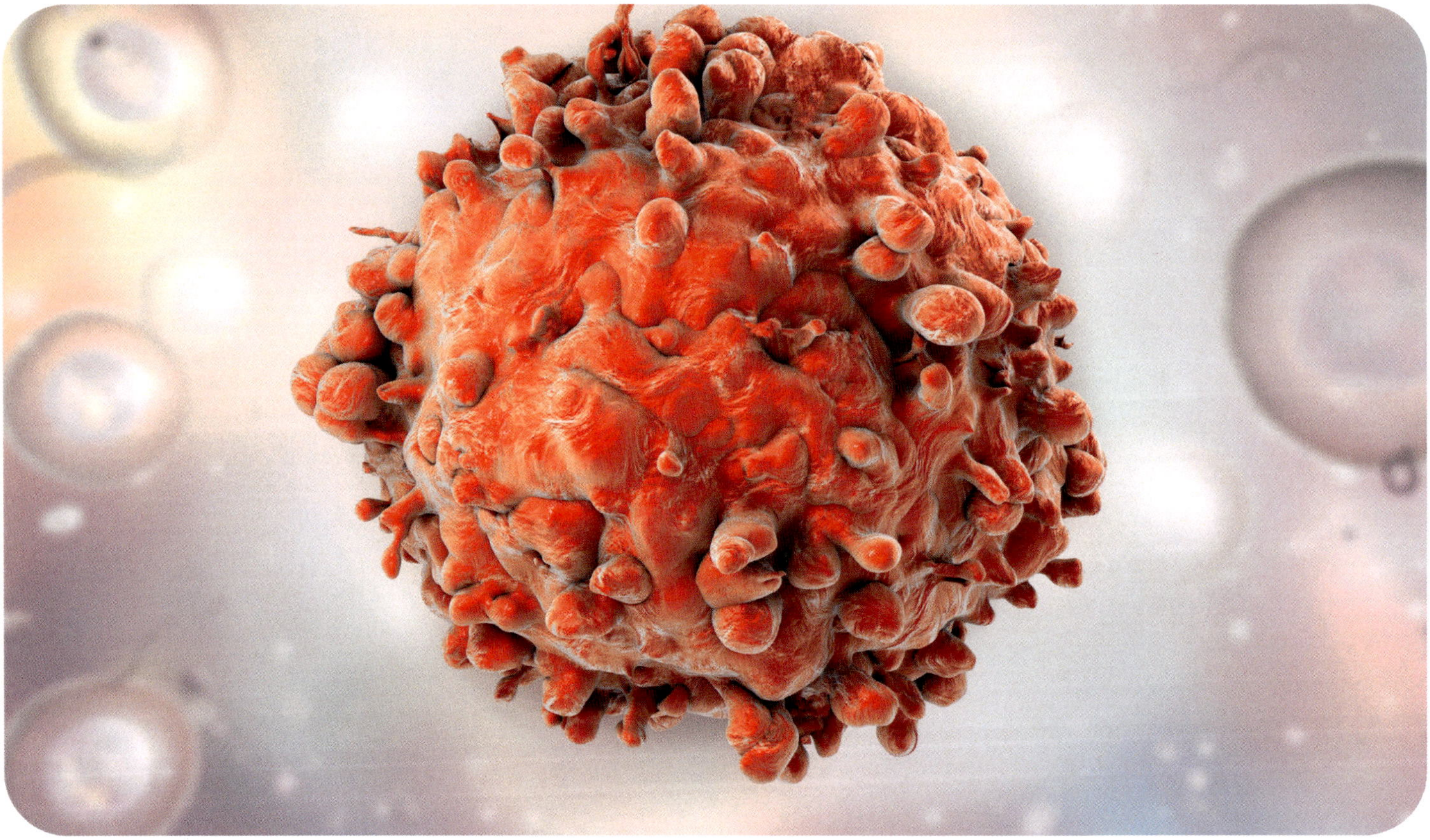

Acute lymphoblastic leukemia (ALL) is a fast-growing cancer that starts in lymphocytes, a type of white blood cell. In ALL, bone marrow makes too many immature lymphocytes called lymphoblasts. Lymphoblasts can crowd out other blood cells causing blood to not work as it should. Treatment depends on the type of ALL, age at diagnosis, and other factors. This book is for those being treated at an adult cancer center.

Blood

Blood is a tissue. A tissue is a group of cells that work together to perform a function. Blood's function is to move oxygen and nutrients throughout your body and carry away waste. Blood also plays an important role for the immune system.

Blood cells

Your blood contains different types of cells that float in plasma. Plasma is a clear, yellowish fluid made up of mostly water. More than half of your blood is plasma.

There are 3 types of blood cells:

- Red blood cells (erythrocytes)
- White blood cells (leukocytes), which include granulocytes, monocytes, and lymphocytes
- Platelets (thrombocytes)

Blood cells have important jobs. Red blood cells carry oxygen throughout the body. White blood cells fight germs. Platelets help control bleeding.

Blood cells are being replaced in your body all the time. Many have a short lifespan. Some white blood cells live less than one day. Your body makes one million red blood cells every second!

Blood stem cells

Bone marrow contains stem cells. A blood stem cell is an immature cell that can develop into a red blood cell, white blood cell, or platelet.

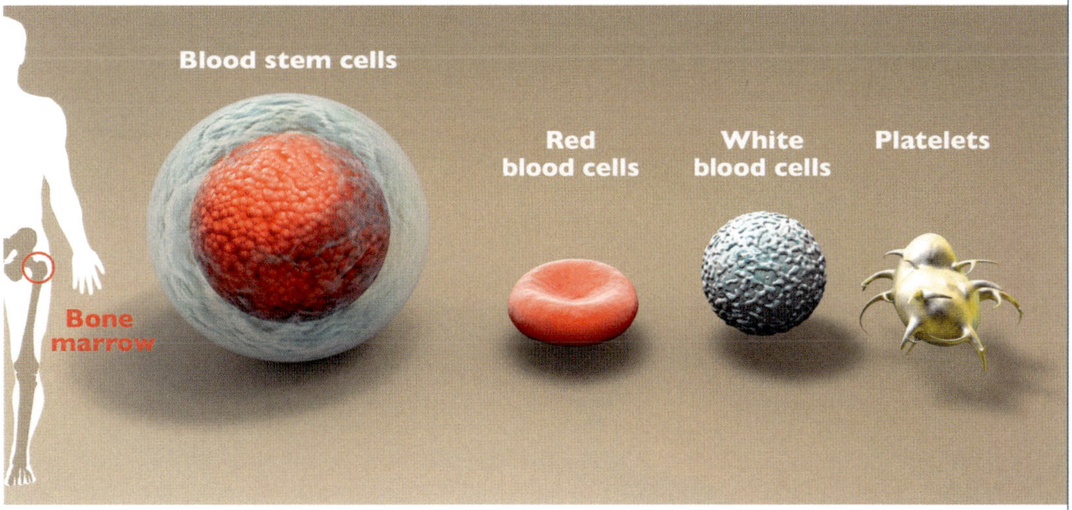

How blood cells are formed

Bone marrow is the sponge-like tissue in the center of most bones. Inside your bone marrow are early blood-forming cells called blood stem cells (hematopoietic stem cells). All types of blood cells start as blood stem cells. At any given time, bone marrow will have cells in various stages of development, from very immature to almost fully mature.

Blood stem cells can do 2 things:

- Make exact copies of themselves
- Make new cells that have the potential to become blood cells

These cells have to mature or go through many stages to become a red blood cell, white blood cell, or platelet. With each stage the blood stem cell changes and gets closer to what it is meant to be. After a blood stem cell develops into a red blood cell, white blood cell, or platelet, it is released in your bloodstream as needed.

Blood stem cells can copy themselves or self-renew. These cells are rare. Blood stem cells can also make new cells that are committed to being a certain type of blood cell. These are called progenitor cells or precursor cells. Progenitor cells are much more common than blood stem cells. Progenitor cells can become red blood cells, white blood cells, or platelets.

Blood cell formation

All blood cells start as blood stem cells. A blood stem cell has to mature or go through many stages to become a red blood cell, white blood cell, or platelet. ALL affects the lymphoid progenitor cells, which develop into a type of white blood cell called lymphocytes.

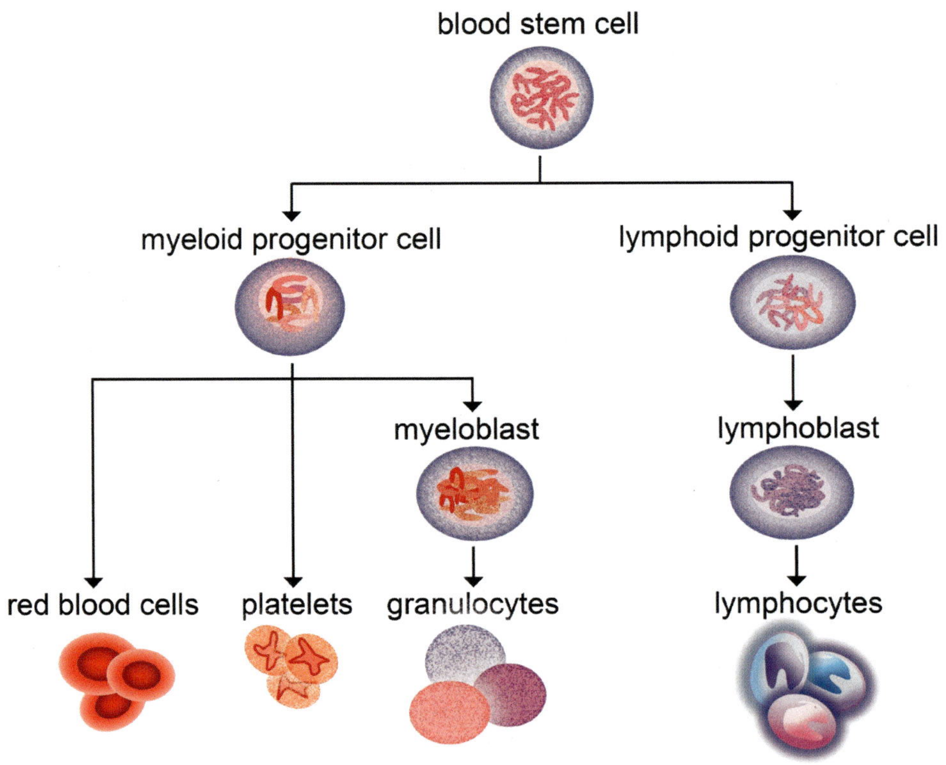

There are 2 types of blood progenitor cells:

- Lymphoid
- Myeloid

Both lymphoid and myeloid progenitor cells form into blast cells called lymphoblasts or myeloblasts depending on the type. Blasts are committed to becoming a type of blood cell. Lymphoblasts are supposed to mature into lymphocytes, a type of white blood cell Lymphoid refers to lymphocyte, a type of white blood cell. Myeloblasts are responsible for all of the other non-lymphoid blood cells in bone marrow.

In acute lymphoblastic leukemia (ALL), lymphoblasts grow out of control in bone marrow. This crowds out blood stems cells and normal red blood cells, platelets, and white blood cells causing blood to not work as it should. The type of ALL depends on the characteristics of the lymphoblasts.

In ALL, lymphoblasts grow out of control in bone marrow causing blood to not work as it should.

Lymphocytes

A lymphocyte is a type of white blood cell. In ALL, bone marrow makes too many immature lymphocytes called lymphoblasts.

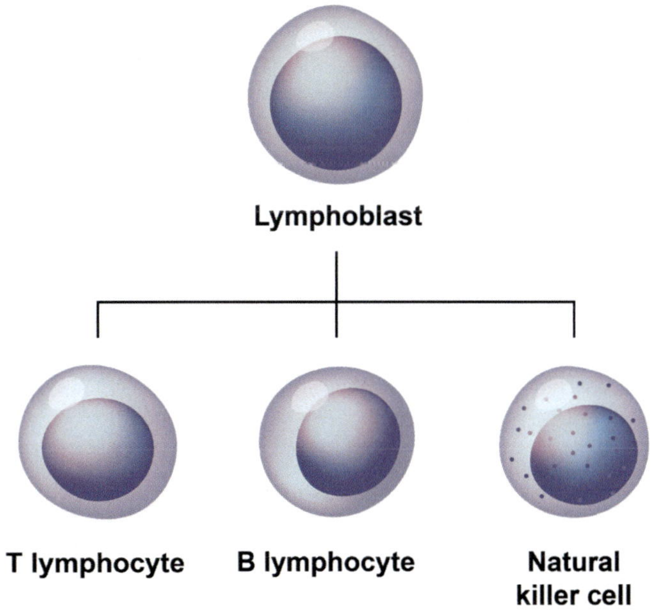

Lymphocytes

A lymphocyte is a type of white blood cell found in blood and lymph tissue. Lymph tissue includes lymph vessels and lymph nodes.

There are 3 main types of lymphocytes:

- B lymphocytes or B cells make antibodies that are used to attack invading bacteria, viruses, and toxins. An antibody is a protein.
- T lymphocytes or T cells are direct fighters of foreign invaders and also produce cytokines, which help activate other parts of the immune system. T cells destroy the body's own cells that have been taken over by viruses or that have become cancerous.
- Natural killer (NK) cells have granules (small particles) with enzymes that can kill tumor cells or cells infected with a virus.

Acute lymphoblastic leukemia

Acute lymphoblastic leukemia (ALL) is a fast-growing blood cancer that starts in disease-fighting lymphocytes of your immune system. In ALL, bone marrow makes too many immature lymphocytes called lymphoblasts. Lymphoblasts can crowd out other blood cells causing blood to not work as it should. Acute leukemias grow faster than chronic leukemias.

ALL most often affects B cells or T cells. To be diagnosed with ALL, 20 percent (20%) or more lymphoblasts must be present in the bone marrow. This means that at least 2 out of every 10 marrow cells are lymphoblasts. In certain cases, a diagnosis of ALL is possible with less than 20% lymphoblasts.

ALL can be found in bone marrow, blood, and organs such as the testicles or the central nervous system (CNS).

ALL diagnosis

To be diagnosed with ALL, 20 percent (20%) or more lymphoblasts must be present in the bone marrow. This means that at least 2 out of every 10 marrow cells are lymphoblasts.

https://commons.wikimedia.org/wiki/File:Acute_lymphoblastic_leukaemia_smear.jpg

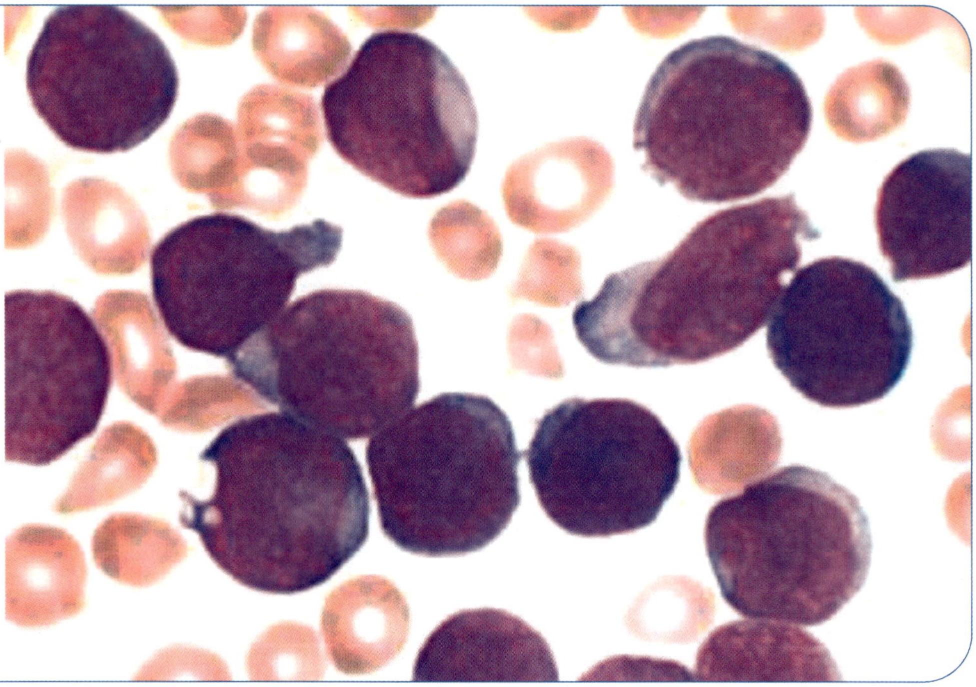

Types of ALL

ALL is a group of diseases. They are grouped and treated based on gene mutations and other features. Genetic testing is very important to identify the ALL subtype. It is a standard part of testing at diagnosis.

There are 2 types of ALL:

- B cell or B-ALL
- T cell or T-ALL

Within each type there are several subtypes, which are based mainly on:

- The type of lymphocyte (most often B cell or T cell) the leukemia cells come from and how mature the cells are. This is known as the immunophenotype of the leukemia.
- If the leukemia cells have certain gene or chromosome changes

B-ALL

B-cell ALL or B-ALL starts in B-cell lymphocytes. B-ALL is more common than T-ALL. Mature B-cell ALL (also called Burkitt leukemia), a rare subtype, is essentially the same as Burkitt lymphoma (a type of non-Hodgkin lymphoma), but is treated differently from B-ALL.

T-ALL

T-cell ALL or T-ALL starts in T-cell lymphocytes. T-ALL can cause an enlarged thymus (a small organ in front of the windpipe), which can sometimes lead to breathing problems.

About this book

This book applies to AYAs and adults who are being treated for ALL at an adult cancer center. An adolescent and young adult (AYA) is someone 15 to 39 years of age at the time of initial cancer diagnosis. AYAs are a unique group that can be treated by pediatric or adult oncologists in pediatric or adult centers depending on the type of cancer.

For AYAs seeking treatment at a pediatric cancer center, see *NCCN Guidelines for Patients: Pediatric Acute Lymphoblastic Leukemia*, available at NCCN.org/patientguidelines.

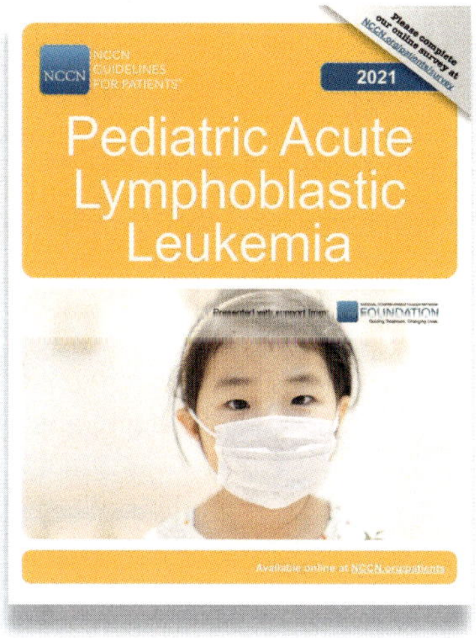

Review

- Acute lymphoblastic leukemia (ALL) is a fast-growing blood cancer. In ALL, bone marrow makes too many immature lymphocytes called lymphoblasts. This makes it hard for blood to do its work.
- To be diagnosed with ALL, 20 percent (20%) or more lymphoblasts must be present in the bone marrow. This means that at least 2 out of every 10 marrow cells are lymphoblasts.
- An adolescent and young adult (AYA) is someone 15 to 39 years of age at the time of initial cancer diagnosis. This book is for AYAs and adults being treated at an adult cancer center.
- There is more than one type of ALL. It is based on the type of lymphocyte, genetic mutations, and other features.
- Those with ALL should be treated at experienced cancer centers.

Those with ALL should be treated at experienced cancer centers.

2

Testing for ALL

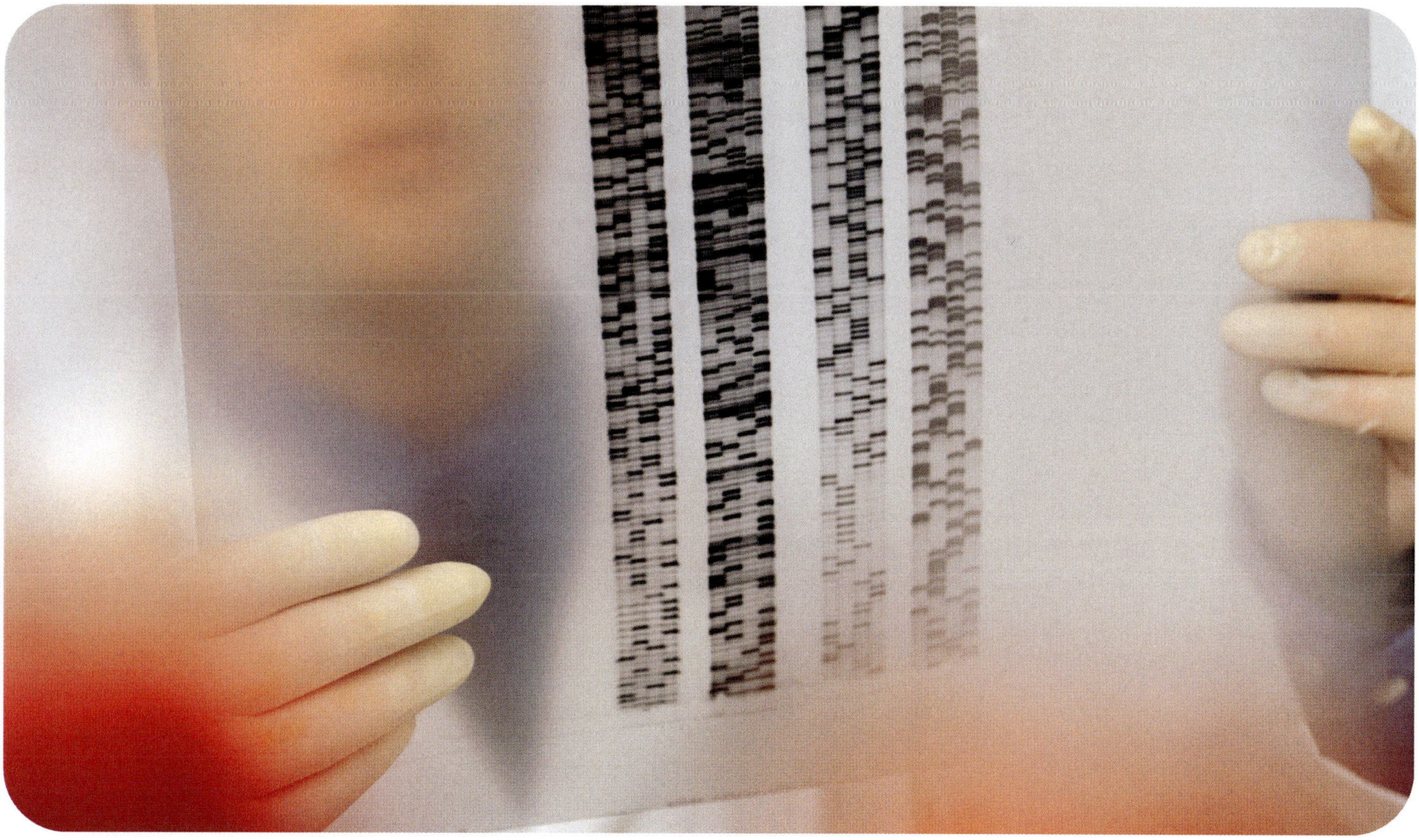

Accurate testing is needed to diagnose and treat ALL. This chapter presents an overview of possible tests and what to expect.

Test results

Test results will determine your treatment plan. It is important you understand what these tests mean. Ask questions and keep copies of your test results. Online patient portals are a great way to access test results.

Whether you are going for a second opinion, test, or office visit, keep these things in mind:

- Bring someone with you to doctor visits, if possible.
- Write down questions and take notes during appointments. Don't be afraid to ask your care team questions. Get to know your care team and let them get to know you.
- Get copies of blood tests, imaging results, and reports about the specific type of cancer you have.
- Organize your papers. Create files for insurance forms, medical records, and test results. You can do the same on your computer.
- Keep a list of contact information for everyone on your care team. Add it to your phone. Hang the list on your fridge or keep it in a place where someone can access it in an emergency.

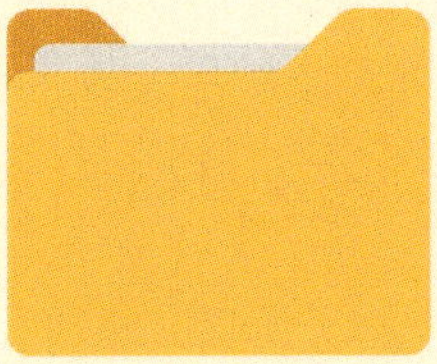

Create a medical binder

A medical binder or notebook is a great way to organize all of your records in one place.

- Make copies of blood tests, imaging results, and reports about your specific type of cancer.
- Choose a binder that meets your needs. Consider a zipper pocket to include a pen, small calendar, and insurance cards.
- Create folders for insurance forms, medical records, and tests results. You can do the same on your computer.
- Use online patient portals to view your test results and other records. Download or print the records to add to your binder.
- Organize your binder in a way that works for you. Add a section for questions and to take notes.
- Bring your medical binder to appointments. You never know when you might need it!

For possible tests, see Guide 1.

Guide 1 Testing for ALL
Medical history and physical exam
Complete blood count (CBC), differential, chemistry profile, liver function tests (LFTs)
Tumor lysis syndrome (TLS) panel: LDH, uric acid, potassium (K), calcium (Ca), phosphorus (Phos)
Disseminated intravascular coagulation (DIC) panel: d-dimer, fibrinogen, prothrombin time (PT), and partial thromboplastin time (PTT)
Testing for hepatitis B and C, HIV, cytomegalovirus (CMV) antibodies (Ab)
Pregnancy testing, fertility counseling, and preservation
CT and MRI of head with contrast, if neurologic symptoms
Lumbar puncture (LP) with intrathecal (IT) chemotherapy
CT of neck, chest, abdomen, pelvis with contrast. PET/CT is possible
Testicular exam, including scrotal ultrasound as needed
Screen for opportunistic infections, as needed
Echocardiogram or cardiac nuclear medicine scan should be considered in all patients
Central venous access device (CVAD) of choice
Strongly consider early transplant evaluation and donor search

General health tests

Medical history

A medical history is a record of all health issues and treatments you have had in your life. Be prepared to list any illness or injury and when it happened. Bring a list of old and new medicines and any over-the-counter medicines, herbals, or supplements you take. Tell your doctor about any symptoms you have. A medical history will help determine which treatment is best for you.

Family history

Some cancers and other diseases can run in families. Your doctor will ask about the health history of family members who are blood relatives. This information is called a family history. Ask family members about their health issues like heart disease, cancer, and diabetes, and at what age they were diagnosed.

Leukemia predisposition syndrome

Certain genetic changes, or mutations, can increase a person's chances of developing cancer. These changes, known as hereditary cancer syndromes, can be passed down from parent to child. Your doctor should do a thorough family history and ask if anyone in your family has had leukemia. If there is a concern for a leukemia predisposition syndrome, you might be referred to a genetic counselor or geneticist. Since family members are often bone marrow donors, it is important to rule out leukemia predisposition syndrome.

Physical exam

A physical exam checks the body for signs of disease.

A health care provider may:

- Check your temperature, blood pressure, pulse, and breathing rate
- Weigh you
- Listen to your lungs and heart
- Look in your eyes, ears, nose, and throat
- Feel and apply pressure to parts of your body to see if organs are of normal size, are soft or hard, or cause pain when touched. Tell your doctor if you feel pain.
- Feel for enlarged lymph nodes in your neck, underarm, and groin. Tell the doctor if you have felt any lumps or have any pain.

Doctors should perform a thorough physical exam along with a complete health history.

Testicular exam

ALL can cause swollen testicles. A testicular exam is a complete physical exam of the groin and the genitals, which are the penis, scrotum, and testicles. Your doctor will feel the organs and check for lumps, swelling, shrinking, and other signs of ALL. Those with testicles should have this exam to look for ALL in this part of the body.

Dental exam

The health of your teeth and gums is important. Some treatments can cause dental problems. Therefore, it is important to see a dentist before and during treatment.

Fertility and birth control

ALL survivors are at risk for fertility issues. Fertility is the ability to have children. In order to preserve one's fertility, action may be needed before starting cancer treatment. However, this is not always possible.

Those who want to have children in the future should be referred to a fertility specialist to discuss the options. More information can be found in *NCCN Guidelines for Patients: Adolescents and Young Adults with Cancer*, available at NCCN.org/patientguidelines.

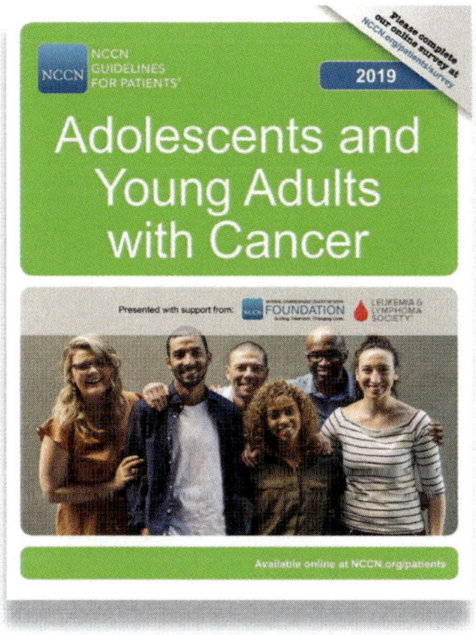

Fertility counseling and preservation options should be presented to everyone with ALL.

Those with ovaries

Those who can have children will have a pregnancy test before starting treatment. Cancer treatment can hurt the baby if you are or become pregnant during treatment. Therefore, birth control to prevent pregnancy during and after treatment is recommended. Hormonal birth control may not be recommended, so ask your doctor about options.

Those with testicles

Cancer and cancer treatment can damage sperm. Therefore, use contraception (birth control) to prevent pregnancy during and after cancer treatment. If you think you want children in the future, talk to your doctor now. Sperm banking may be an option.

Infertility

Infertility is the complete loss of the ability to have children. The actual risk of infertility is related to your age at time of diagnosis, treatment type(s), treatment dose, and treatment length. Chemotherapy with alkylating agents has a higher risk of infertility. Sometimes, there isn't time for fertility preservation before you start treatment. Talk to your doctor about your concerns.

Blood tests

Blood tests check for signs of disease and how well organs are working. They require a sample of blood, which is removed through a needle placed into your vein.

Pregnancy test

Those who can become pregnant will be given a pregnancy test before treatment begins.

Complete blood count

A complete blood count (CBC) measures the levels of red blood cells, white blood cells, and platelets in your blood. Red blood cells carry oxygen throughout your body, white blood cells fight infection, and platelets control bleeding.

Differential

There are 5 types of white blood cells: neutrophils, lymphocytes, monocytes, eosinophils, and basophils. A differential counts the number of each type of white blood cell (WBC). It also checks if the counts are in balance with each other.

Chemistry profile

A chemistry profile or panel measures different substances in your blood. The liver, bone, and other organs release chemicals in your blood. A chemistry profile measures these levels.

CMV Ab

Cytomegalovirus (CMV) Ab testing looks for antibodies to CMV, a virus in the herpes family. CMV is very common. Most people do not even know they have it.

Be prepared to have a lot of blood tests.

Hepatitis B and C

Hepatitis is a virus that causes inflammation of the liver. Hepatitis B (HBV) and hepatitis C (HCV) are spread by contact with blood and other bodily fluids. A blood test will show if you had hepatitis in the past or if you have it today. Treatment with immunotherapy and chemotherapy might cause hepatitis B to reactivate, which can cause liver damage.

HIV

Human immunodeficiency virus (HIV) causes acquired immunodeficiency syndrome (AIDS). An HIV antibody test checks for HIV antibodies in a sample of blood, urine, or saliva.

Liver function tests

Liver function tests (LFTs) look at the health of your liver by measuring chemicals that are made or processed by the liver. Levels that are too high or low signal that the liver is not working well or the bile ducts might be blocked.

Opportunistic infections

Opportunistic infections (OIs) are infections that occur more frequently and are more severe in those with a weakened immune system. Drug treatment for ALL can weaken the body's natural defense against infections. You will be monitored for OIs, as needed.

If not treated early, infections can be fatal. Infections can be caused by viruses, fungus, or bacteria. Antibiotics can treat bacterial infections. Antifungal medicines can treat fungal infections. You may be given antiviral drugs to prevent viral infections.

Blood clotting tests

Your body stops bleeding by turning blood into a gel-like form. The gel-like blood forms into a solid mass called a blood clot. Clotting is a process or series of events. Proteins, called coagulation factors, are needed for clotting. They are made by the liver. These tests are known together as a coagulation panel or disseminated intravascular coagulation (DIC) panel.

A DIC panel includes:

- D-dimer is present when the body is forming and breaking down blood clots. Prothrombin time (PT) and partial thromboplastin time (PTT) measure how long it takes blood to clot.
- Fibrinogen activity measures how much fibrinogen, a blood protein, is being made by the liver.

An impaired clotting process is common in leukemia. This is called coagulopathy. You may have bleeding and bruises or blood clots. It is standard to screen for clotting problems.

Tumor lysis syndrome panel

Cancer treatment causes cell death. In tumor lysis syndrome (TLS), waste released by dead cells builds up in the body causing kidney damage and severe blood electrolyte disturbances.

If you are at risk for TLS, you will have blood tests daily. Changes in creatinine, lactic acid, uric acid, phosphorus (Phos), potassium (K), and calcium (Ca) levels can be sign of TLS.

Creatinine

Creatinine is a waste produced in the muscles. It is filtered out of the blood by the kidneys and tells how well the kidneys are working.

Lactic acid

Lactate dehydrogenase (LDH) or lactic acid dehydrogenase is a protein found in most cells. Dying cells release LDH into blood. Fast-growing cells also release LDH. High levels of LDH can be a sign of ALL.

Uric acid

Uric acid is released by cells when DNA breaks down. It is a normal waste product that dissolves in your blood and is filtered by the kidneys where it leaves the body as urine. Too much uric acid in the body is called hyperuricemia. With ALL, it can be caused by a fast turnover of white blood cells. High uric acid might be a side effect of chemotherapy or radiation therapy.

Lumbar puncture

A lumbar puncture (LP) or spinal tap is a procedure that removes spinal fluid. It is also used to inject chemotherapy into the spinal fluid. This is called intrathecal (IT) chemotherapy.

At the time of IT, a sample of your spinal fluid will be taken and tested. Leukemia can travel to the cerebrospinal fluid (CSF) that surrounds the spine or brain. This is called central nervous system (CNS) disease. Systemic therapy and IT therapy are given together to prevent CNS disease. This is called CNS prophylaxis. IT therapy needs to be given even if the CNS is negative because leukemia is likely to return here.

Tissue tests

A biopsy is needed to diagnose ALL. A biopsy is the removal of a sample of tissue or group of cells for testing. Your sample should be reviewed by a pathologist who is an expert in the diagnosis of ALL. This review is often referred to as histology or histopathology review. The pathologist will note the overall appearance and the size, shape, and type of your cells.

Tissue and cells removed during a biopsy will be tested.

Lumbar puncture

A lumbar puncture is a procedure that removes spinal fluid.

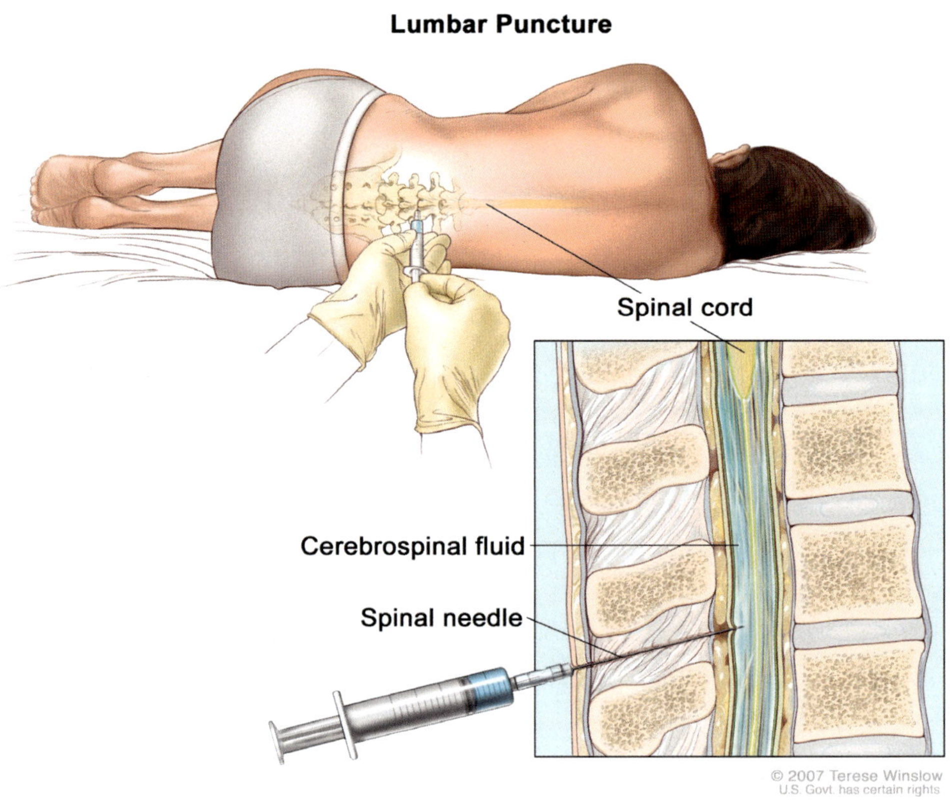

Bone marrow tests

Leukemia starts in the bone marrow. To diagnose ALL, samples of bone marrow must be removed. Lab results will be used to confirm the disease. Your bone marrow will also be tested to see how well treatment is working.

There are 2 types of bone marrow tests that are often done at the same time:

- Bone marrow aspirate
- Bone marrow biopsy

Your bone marrow is like a sponge holding liquid and cells. An aspirate takes some of the liquid and cells out of the sponge, and a biopsy takes a piece of the sponge.

The samples are usually taken from the back of the hip bone (pelvis). You will likely lie on your belly or side. Your doctors will first clean and give sedation or numb your skin and outer surface of your bone. For an aspirate, a hollow needle will be pushed through your skin and into the bone. Liquid bone marrow will then be drawn into a syringe. For the biopsy, a wider needle will be used to remove a core sample. You may feel bone pain at your hip for a few days. Your skin may bruise.

Bone marrow biopsy

Samples of bone and marrow are removed in a biopsy.

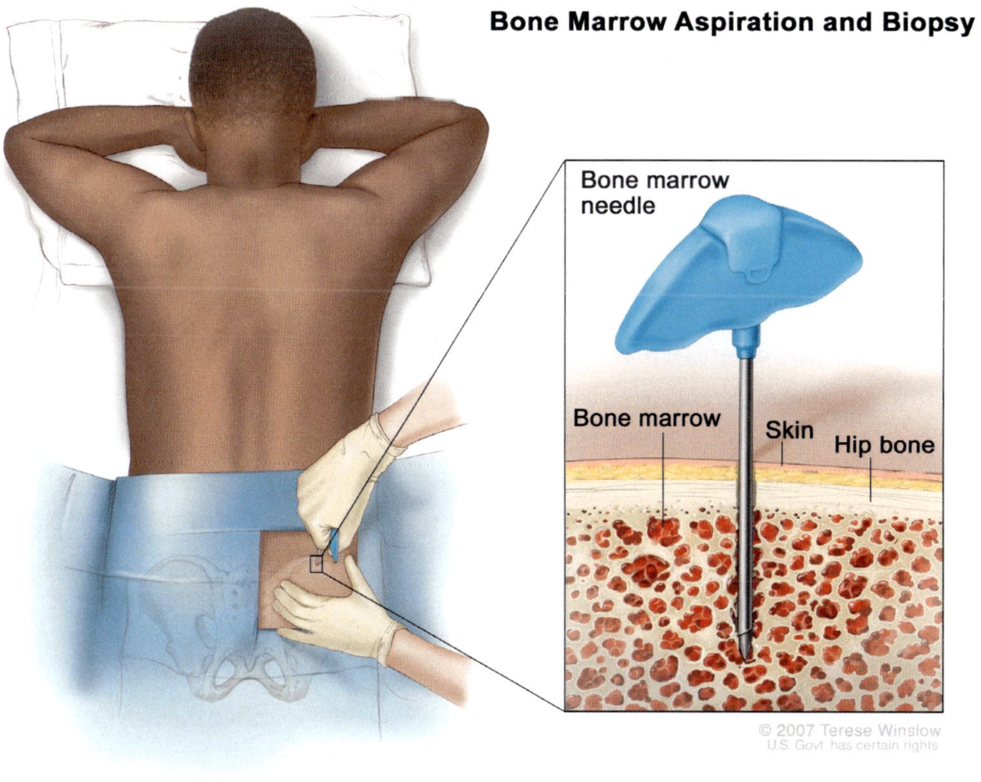

Skin punch biopsy

If a predisposition syndrome is suspected, you might have a skin punch biopsy. Genetic testing for leukemia can't be done using blood or saliva. If you tested the blood at diagnosis, you would see the genetic changes of the leukemia. Therefore, a skin punch biopsy is used. In this procedure, a small piece of skin and connective tissue are removed to get DNA that hasn't been altered by ALL. This will be used to see if you have inherited genes that increase your risk of leukemia. Leukemia predisposition syndrome can affect how your body responds to treatment.

Flow cytometry

Flow cytometry is a laboratory method used to detect, identify, and count specific cells. Flow cytometry involves adding a light-sensitive dye to cells. The dyed cells are passed through a beam of light in a machine. The machine measures the number of cells, things like the size and shape of the cells, and proteins on the surface of thousands of cells.

Flow cytometry may be used on cells from circulating (peripheral) blood, bone marrow, or a biopsy. The most common use of flow cytometry is in the identification of markers on cells, particularly in the immune system (called immunophenotyping). Treatments can target these specific antigens or proteins on the surface of the leukemia cells, including CD19, CD20, and CD22.

A blood test can count the number of white blood cells, but it cannot detect the subtle differences between different types of blood cancers. Flow cytometry can detect these subtle differences. This test is important because the immunophenotype may affect which treatment is best for you.

Immunophenotyping

Immunophenotyping uses antibodies to detect the presence or absence of white blood cell antigens. These antigens are proteins that can be found on the surface of or inside white blood cells. They are called markers or biomarkers. Certain biomarkers such as CD19, CD20, and CD22 are targeted in ALL treatment.

Immunophenotyping is done using flow cytometry. It is used to pinpoint the type of ALL. Immunophenotype can change as cancer progresses.

Based on immunophenotype, ALL can be placed into 2 general groups:

- B-cell ALL
- T-cell ALL

B-ALL

B-ALL is the most common type of ALL. It starts in immature cells (lymphoblasts) that would normally develop into B lymphocytes. Subtypes include early precursor B cell (early pre-B cell) and pre-B cell. Mature B-cell ALL (Burkitt lymphoma) is a rare subtype. B-ALL can be Philadelphia chromosome-positive (Ph+) or Philadelphia chromosome-negative (Ph-).

T-ALL

T-ALL starts in lymphoblasts that would normally develop into T-cell lymphocytes. This type is less common, and it occurs more often in adolescent boys. A protein called CD3 is typically found in T-ALL. Others may be present. T-ALL does not have the Philadelphia chromosome (Ph-). Early T-cell precursor (ETP-ALL) is a distinct subtype of T-ALL.

Genetic tests

Genetic tests are used to learn more about your type of ALL, to target treatment, and to determine the likely path your cancer will take (prognosis).

Inside our cells are deoxyribonucleic acid (DNA) molecules. These molecules are tightly packaged into what is called a chromosome. Chromosomes contain most of the genetic information in a cell. Normal human cells contain 23 pairs of chromosomes for a total of 46 chromosomes. Each chromosome contains thousands of genes. Genes tell cells what to do and what to become.

ALL can cause changes in genes and chromosomes in blood cells. Genetic tests look for these changes or abnormalities. You may be placed into a risk group based on the types of genetic abnormalities found.

Comparative genomic hybridization

Comparative genomic hybridization (CGH) is a technique that compares DNA samples from normal tissue and tumor tissue. It is used to detect abnormal chromosomes.

High-throughput sequencing

High-throughput sequencing (HTS) is capable of sequencing hundreds of millions of DNA molecules at a time.

Next-generation sequencing

Next-generation sequencing (NGS) is a high-throughput method used to determine a portion of a person's DNA sequence.

FISH

Fluorescence in situ hybridization (FISH) is a method that involves special dyes called probes that attach to pieces of DNA. For example, the probes attach to the *BCR* gene and the *ABL* gene. The *BCR-ABL1* gene is detected when the colors of the probes overlap by translocation. A translocation is the switching of parts between two chromosomes. Another possible translocation found in ALL is *KMT2A* or t(v;11q23.3). FISH can look for other translocations that are too small to be seen with other methods.

Since this test doesn't need growing cells, it can be performed on either a bone marrow or blood sample. However, FISH can only be used for known changes. It cannot detect all the possible changes found with a karyotype. Sometimes, a bone marrow sample will still be needed to get all of the information your doctor needs to help plan your care.

Karyotype

A karyotype is a picture of chromosomes. Doctors look for whether 46 chromosomes or 23 pairs are present. They also look for extra, missing, or abnormal pieces of chromosomes, such as the *BCR-ABL1* gene. Since a karyotype requires growing cells, a sample of bone marrow must be used.

PCR

A polymerase chain reaction (PCR) is a lab process that can make millions or billions of copies of your DNA (genetic information). PCR is very sensitive. It can find 1 leukemia cell among more than 100,000 normal cells.

A special PCR called quantitative reverse transcriptase-polymerase chain reaction (qPCR) measures the number of cells with the *BCR-ABL1* gene. This test might be referred to as real-time or reverse transcriptase (RT) PCR.

A bone marrow biopsy is needed to diagnose ALL.

ALL mutation testing

Cells in your body contain chromosomes. Chromosomes are long strands of genetic information called DNA (deoxyribonucleic acid). Your DNA uses coded instructions to tell your cells what to do. These instructions are called genes.

Cancer starts when something goes wrong in the DNA of a cell. Abnormal changes in the genes of cancer cells are possible. These abnormal changes are called mutations. Mutations are often found in ALL. ALL can change the DNA in your blood cells.

Karyotype

A karyotype is a picture of your chromosomes.

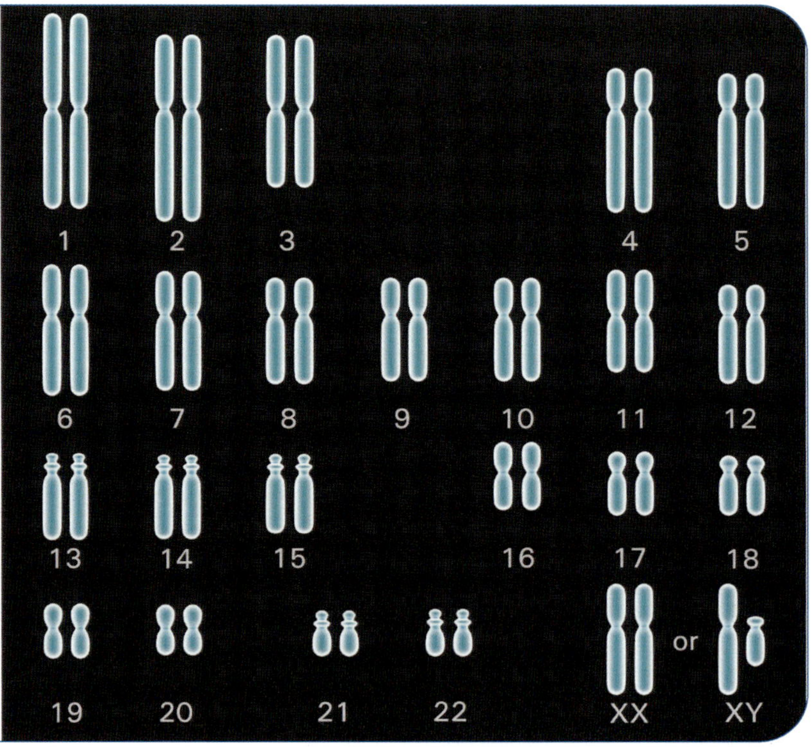

A sample of your blood or bone marrow will be used to see if ALL cancer cells have any specific mutations. Some mutations can be targeted with specific therapies. This is separate from the genetic testing for mutations that you may have inherited from your parents.

For a list of some of the genetic abnormalities found in ALL, see Guide 2.

Guide 2
A list of some gene or chromosome changes found in ALL

B-ALL	Hyperdiploidy (leukemia cells with more than 50 chromosomes)
	Hypodiploidy (leukemia cells with fewer than 44 chromosomes)
	t(9;22)(q34;q11) translocation that results in *BCR-ABL1*
	t(12;21)(p13;q22) translocation that results in *ETV6-RUNX1*
	t(v;11q23) translocation that results in *KMT2A rearranged*
	t(1;19)(q23;p13) translocation that results in *TCF3-PBX1*
	t(5;14)(q31;q32) translocation that results in *IL3-IGH*
	t(8;14), t(2;8), t(8;22) translocations that result in *c-MYC*
	t(11;14)(q11) translocation that results in *TCRα* and *TCRδ*
	Ikaros translocation that results in *IKZF1*
	B-lymphoblastic leukemia/lymphoma with translocations involving tyrosine kinases or cytokine receptors (also known as *BCR-ABL1*–like ALL or Ph-like ALL)
	B-lymphoblastic leukemia/lymphoma with intrachromosomal amplification (too many copies) of a portion of chromosome 21 (*iAMP21*)
T-ALL	t(1;14)(p32;q11) translocation that results in *TAL-1*
	t(10;14)(q24;q11) translocation that results in *HOX11 (TLX1)*
	t(5;14)(q35;q32) translocation that results in *HOX11L2*

Philadelphia chromosome

All cells in our body contain genetic information organized in chromosomes. A cell must make a copy of its chromosomes before dividing into two cells. Sometimes, there are mistakes in the copies. One type of mistake is when parts of two chromosomes break off and switch with each other. This is called a translocation. It can result in a fusion gene. There are a few different translocations that might be found in ALL. One is the Philadelphia chromosome (Ph).

In the Philadelphia chromosome, a piece of chromosome 9 and a piece of chromosome 22 break off and trade places with each other. These pieces then fuse together on chromosome 22. This new, abnormal chromosome 22 is referred to as the Philadelphia chromosome. You might see it written as Ph-positive (Ph+).

The piece of chromosome 9 is a gene called *ABL*. The piece of chromosome 22 is a gene called *BCR*. When these genes fuse together on chromosome 22, the *BCR-ABL1* gene is formed. *BCR-ABL1* is a fusion gene. It is not found in normal blood cells. It is not passed down from parents to children.

BCR-ABL1 makes a new protein that leads to uncontrolled cell growth. Treatment for Ph+ ALL aims to stop the activity of the *BCR-ABL* fusion protein. Genes are written like this: *BCR-ABL*. Proteins are written like this: BCR-ABL.

Philadelphia chromosome

The Philadelphia chromosome is formed by a translocation between parts of chromosomes 9 and 22. It contains the abnormal *BCR-ABL1* fusion gene.

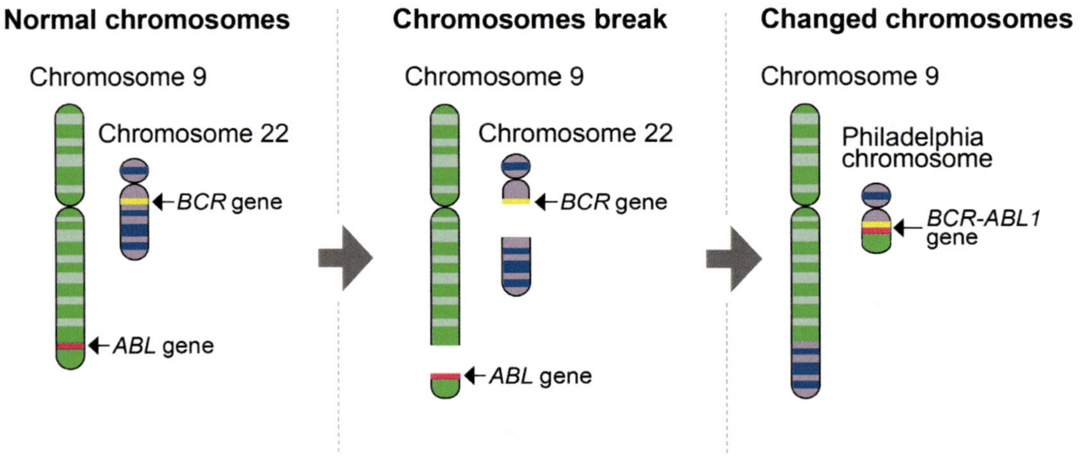

B-ALL genetic risk groups

Some genetic mutations respond better to treatment and are labeled "good risk." Poor risk mutations are more of a challenge to treat. For B-ALL genetic risk groups, see Guide 3.

Genetic risk factors include:

- Hypodiploidy or hyperdiploidy
- Gene or chromosome mutations

Testing lymphoblasts in bone marrow or blood for specific genetic abnormalities is an important part of treatment planning.

Guide 3
Genetic risk groups for B-ALL

Good risk	High hyperdiploidy (leukemia cells have 51 to 65 chromosomes) • Trisomy of chromosomes 4, 10, and 17 are among trisomies that have the most favorable outcome
	t(12;21)(p13;q22): *ETV6-RUNX1*
Poor risk	Hypodiploidy (leukemia cells have fewer than 44 chromosomes)
	KMT2A rearranged
	t(v;14q32)/IgH
	t(9;22)(q34;q11.2): *BCR-ABL1*
	Complex karyotype (5 or more chromosomal abnormalities)
	BCR-ABL1-like (Ph-like) ALL • JAK-STAT (*CRLF2r, EPORr, JAK1/2/3r, TYK2r,* mutations of *SH2B3, IL7R, JAK1/2/3*) • ABL class (rearrangements of *ABL1, ABL2, PDGFRA, PDGFRB, FGFR*) • Other *(NTRKr, FLT3r, LYNr, PTL2Br)*
	Intrachromosomal amplification of chromosome 21 (*iAMP21)*
	t(17;19): *TCF3-HLF* fusion
	Alterations of *IKZF1*

Other factors that might impact treatment include:

- Predisposition syndrome
- Down syndrome
- Age
- White blood cell (WBC) count at diagnosis
- Presence of central nervous system (CNS) disease
- Response to induction (first) treatment
- If minimal residual disease (MRD) remains after treatment

Hypodiploidy

In hypodiploidy, leukemia cells have fewer than 44 chromosomes. Normal cells have 46 chromosomes.

Hyperdiploidy

In hyperdiploidy, leukemia cells have more than 50 chromosomes. Normal cells have 46 chromosomes.

Age

As the body ages, it can have difficulty tolerating higher doses or more intense cancer treatments. Your overall health and general level of fitness, called performance status, also play a role in treatment decisions.

WBC

A WBC of 30 x 10^9/L or higher for B lineage or 100 x 10^9/L or higher for T lineage at initial diagnosis is sometimes considered high risk.

Down syndrome

In Down syndrome or trisomy 21, there is an extra chromosome 21. Instead of two chromosomes, there are three (called trisomy). There are challenges treating those with Down syndrome.

Predisposition syndrome

Some hereditary cancer syndromes can be passed down from parent to child. A family history of leukemia can affect treatment.

BCR-ABL1-like (Ph-like) ALL

Ph-like B-ALL does not have the Philadelphia chromosome (Ph-). Tests will look for specific genetic fusions and mutations to confirm a diagnosis of Ph-like ALL. Ph-like ALL is difficult to treat due to the number of possible mutations. It might be referred to as *BCR-ABL1*-like ALL. If you have Ph-like ALL talk to your doctor about which treatment options might be right for you.

Heart tests

Certain treatments can affect cardiac function. Heart or cardiac tests are used to see how well your heart works. These tests might be used as a baseline and before giving chemotherapy. You might be referred to a cardiologist.

Echocardiogram

An echocardiogram (or echo) uses sound waves to make pictures. For this test, small patches will be placed on your chest to track your heartbeat. Next, a wand with gel on its tip will be slid across part of your bare chest. A picture of your beating heart will be seen on a screen. The pictures will be recorded for future viewing.

An echocardiogram is one way of measuring ejection fraction, which is the amount of blood pumped out of the left side of your heart every time it beats. In low ejection fraction, the amount of blood pumping from the left side of the heart is lower than normal.

Cardiac nuclear medicine scan

A nuclear heart scan is an imaging test that uses special cameras and a radioactive substance called a tracer to create pictures of your heart. The tracer is injected into your blood and travels to your heart.

Echocardiogram

An echocardiogram is one way of measuring ejection fraction, which is the amount of blood pumped out of the left side of your heart each time it beats. Measurement of ejection fraction is recommended for most people before starting some types of chemotherapy.

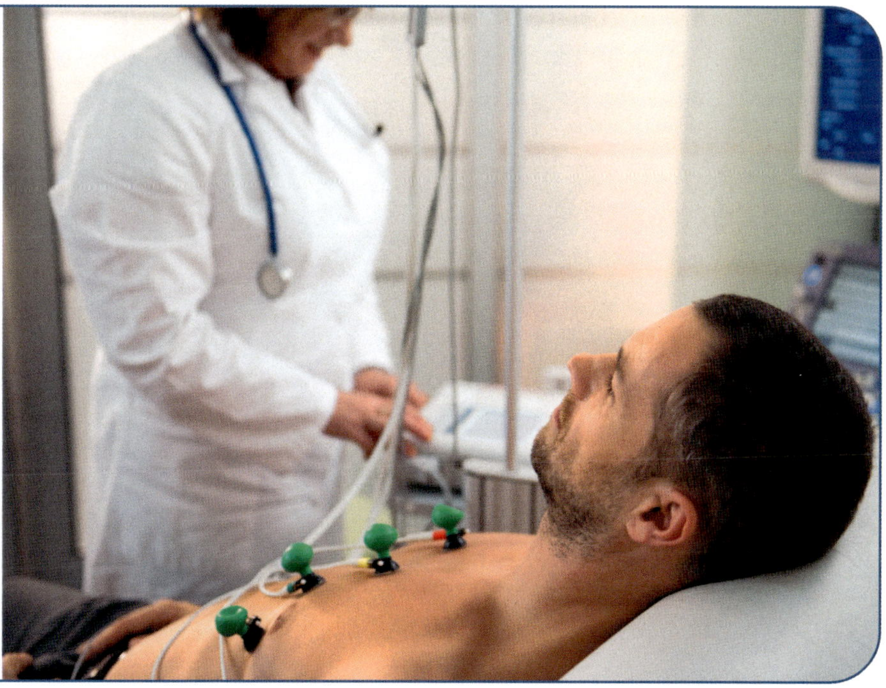

Imaging tests

Imaging tests take pictures (images) of the inside of your body. These tests are used to look for cancer in organs and areas outside of the blood. A radiologist, an expert in test images, will write a report and send this report to your doctor. Your doctor will discuss the results with you.

Chest x-ray

An x-ray is a type of radiation. In small doses, it is used to make pictures of the inside of the body.

CT scan

A computed tomography (CT or CAT) scan uses x-rays and computer technology to take pictures of the inside of the body. It takes many x-rays of the same body part from different angles. All the images are combined to make one detailed picture. In most cases, contrast will be used. Contrast materials are not dyes, but substances that help certain areas in the body stand out. They are used to make the pictures clearer. Contrast materials are not permanent and will leave the body in your urine.

Tell your doctors if you have had bad reactions to contrast in the past. This is important. You might be given medicines, such as Benadryl® and prednisone, for an allergy to contrast. Contrast might not be used if you have a serious allergy or if your kidneys aren't working well.

MRI scan

A magnetic resonance imaging (MRI) scan uses radio waves and powerful magnets to take pictures of the inside of the body. It does not use x-rays. Contrast might be used. Since ALL has risk for spreading to the central nervous system, an MRI of the brain and spinal cord might be done.

PET scan

A positron emission tomography (PET) scan uses a radioactive drug called a tracer. A tracer is a substance injected into a vein to see where it is in the body and if it is using sugar to grow. Cancer cells show up as bright spots on PET scans. Not all bright spots are cancer. It is normal for the brain, heart, kidneys, and bladder to be bright on PET. When a PET scan is combined with CT, it is called a PET/CT scan. PET may be done if there is concern ALL is present outside of the bone marrow.

Scrotal ultrasound

A scrotal ultrasound uses sound waves to make images of the scrotum. The scrotum is the pouch of skin at the base of the penis that contains the testicles. The images are recorded on a computer. There is a higher risk of ALL going to this part of the body.

Review

- Results from blood and tissue tests, imaging studies, and biopsy will determine the treatment plan.
- A biopsy is the removal of a sample of tissue or group of cells for testing. A diagnosis of ALL is confirmed using either a bone marrow aspirate or bone marrow biopsy.
- Immunophenotyping is used to pinpoint the type of ALL.
- You may might be placed into a risk group before starting treatment. Risk might be reassessed between stages of treatment.
- Factors that can affect treatment include age, white blood cell count at diagnosis, predisposition syndrome, Down syndrome, and gene or chromosome mutations.
- Cancer treatment can affect fertility.
- Blood tests check for signs of disease, how well organs are working, and treatment results. Blood clotting tests will also be done.
- Imaging tests are used to look for sites of infection, bleeding, and leukemia that might have spread outside the bloodstream.
- Heart or cardiac tests are used to see how well your heart works. These tests might be used to monitor treatment side effects.
- Leukemia can travel to the cerebrospinal fluid (CSF) that surrounds the spine or brain. It can also travel to sites outside of the blood such as the testicles.

3
Treatment phases

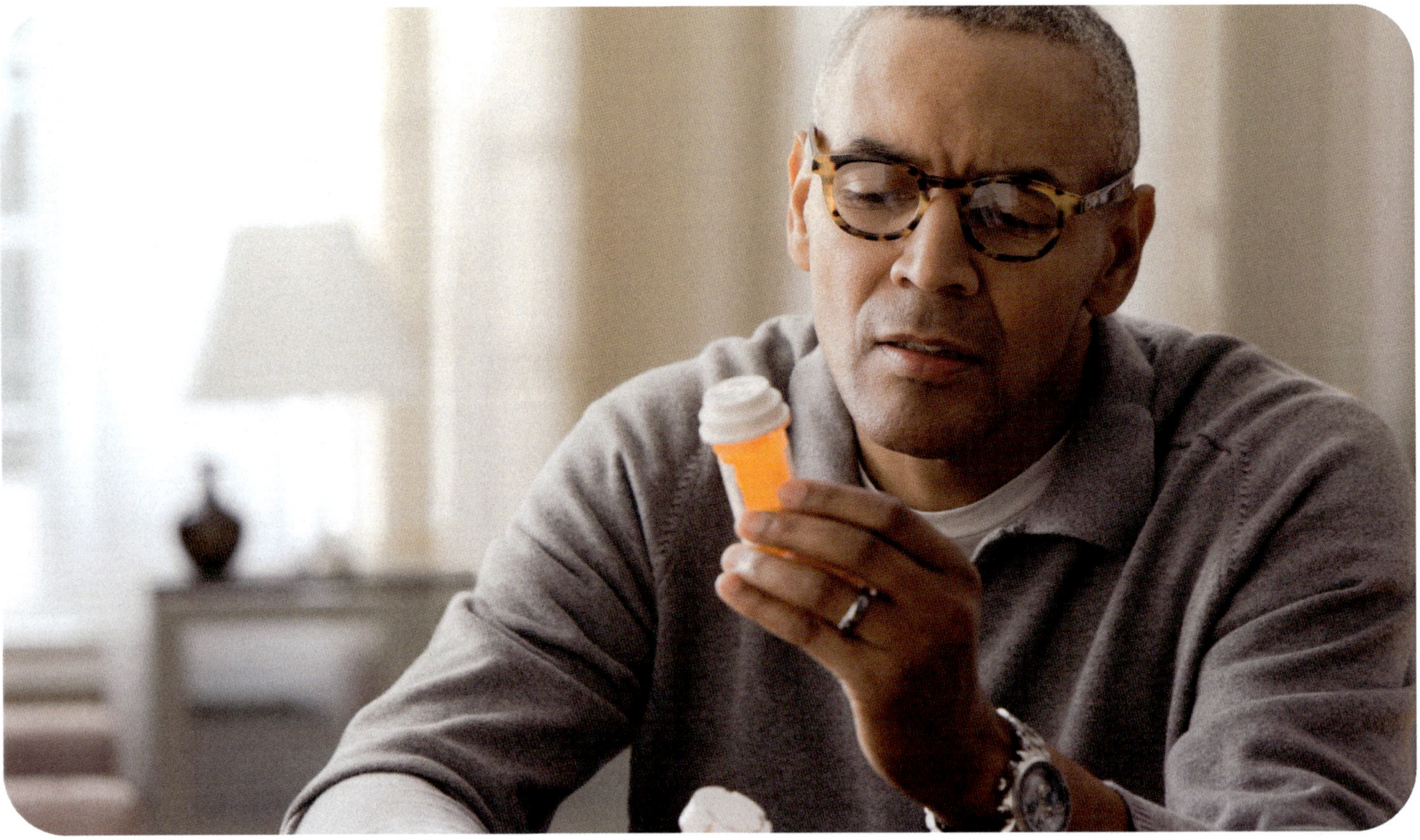

The goal of treatment is a complete response or complete remission. Treatment will be in phases. The three phases of treatment are induction, consolidation, and maintenance.

In an incomplete blood count recovery (CRi), the platelet count or absolute neutrophil count (ANC) has not yet returned to normal. ANC is an estimate of the body's ability to fight infections, especially bacterial infections.

Types of response

There are different types of treatment response. When there are no signs of cancer, it is called a complete response (CR) or complete remission. This does not always mean that ALL has been cured. Remission can be short-term (temporary) or long-lasting (permanent).

A diagnosis of ALL is based on the presence of 20 percent (20%) or more lymphoblasts in the bone marrow. This means that at least 2 out of every 10 marrow cells are lymphoblasts. However, in some cases a diagnosis of ALL is possible with less than 20% blasts. Treatment aims to reduce the number of blasts.

In complete response all of the following are true:

- Absolute neutrophil count (ANC) is more than 1,000/µL
- Platelet count is more than 100,000/µL
- No lymphoblasts are found in blood
- Less than 5% blasts are found in bone marrow (or fewer than 5 blasts out of every 100 blood cells)
- No signs and symptoms of cancer outside the bone marrow (extramedullary disease)
- Cancer has not returned in 4 weeks

Phases of treatment

There are 3 phases of treatment: induction, consolidation, and maintenance. However, not all doctors use the same terms when discussing treatment. In general, there are several phases of intense chemotherapy followed by a longer phase of maintenance chemotherapy. The number of phases and the type chemotherapy given depends on the type of leukemia, as well as how you respond to the first phases of treatment.

Induction

Induction is the first phase of treatment. You will likely spend time in the hospital for part of this treatment. Treatment is a multi-drug combination of chemotherapies (called multi-agent chemotherapy) and steroids.

The goal of induction is a complete response (CR) or remission. In CR, less than 5% blasts remain at the end of induction. This is measured using a microscope and a sample of your bone marrow. When less than 5% blasts remain, the bone marrow can return to normal function. However, leukemia cells may remain in the body. This is called minimal or measurable residual disease (MRD).

When induction does not lead to a CR, it is called induction failure. This could be a sign that this cancer is very difficult to treat. How the cancer responds to initial treatment affects prognosis. Treatment following induction failure is often an allogeneic stem cell transplant (allo-SCT). However, a different multi-agent chemotherapy might be tried before an SCT in order to reduce the amount of MRD.

Minimal residual disease

After induction, you will have bone marrow tests to look for a complete response and to measure the amount of cancer that might remain MRD. More sensitive means than a microscope will be used to look for MRD.

In MRD, ALL is detected in your bone marrow using flow cytometry or PCR. Not all MRD can be found with tests. The aim of treatment will be to reduce the amount of MRD.

What do I need to know?

Seek out support groups at your local hospital, through social media, or from those listed in the back of this book. Look to friends, relatives, neighbors, and co-workers for social support. AYAs also need a support network. Their network might look different than yours. Support services such as counseling are also available. Ask the treatment team for more information. They are there to help.

Consolidation

Consolidation is the second phase of treatment. It is needed to kill any cancer cells that might remain after induction.

Consolidation lasts 6 to 9 months and aims to prevent cancer from returning. The time spent in consolidation and the intensity of the drug regimen will vary. It will be based on factors such as your age, how well you respond to treatment, and risk factors.

It is very important to take medicine on time and exactly as prescribed. Don't miss or skip a dose!

Maintenance

Maintenance chemotherapy is the final, and longest, stage of treatment ALL. Treatment is less intensive than prior chemotherapy. It usually lasts at least 2 years and is outpatient. The goal is to lower the risk of relapse.

What do I need to know?

It is very important to continue to take your medicine as prescribed and not miss or skip any doses. This helps to prevent relapse. Ask your treatment team for help if you have trouble paying for medicine or trouble remembering to take your medicine.

Prevention and treatment of CNS disease

Treatment to prevent ALL from spreading to the central nervous system (CNS) is called CNS prophylaxis or prophylactic treatment. CNS prophylaxis is typically given throughout the entire course of ALL therapy, from induction, to consolidation, to the maintenance phases of treatment.

All treatment plans include intrathecal (IT) chemotherapy. IT chemotherapy is injected into spinal fluid. Some treatments include intrathecal treatment throughout therapy, whereas others do not include it in maintenance. Options for intrathecal chemotherapy include intrathecal methotrexate or a combination of intrathecal methotrexate, cytarabine, and hydrocortisone (known as triple intrathecal chemotherapy).

Treatment is needed to prevent ALL from spreading to the central nervous system (CNS). This is called CNS prophylaxis.

CNS relapse

Sometimes ALL travels to or relapses in the CNS. In this case, special treatment is needed. Treatment of CNS disease includes systemic chemotherapy able to penetrate the blood-brain barrier, direct intrathecal chemotherapy, and cranial irradiation.

Surveillance and monitoring

Monitoring or surveillance watches for any changes in your condition.

For a list and timing of the tests your might receive, see Guide 4.

Guide 4
Surveillance and monitoring

Surveillance	1 year after treatment →	Every 1 to 2 months • Physical exam • CBC with differential • LFTs until normal
	2 years after treatment →	Every 3 to 6 months • Physical exam • CBC with differential
	3 years or more after treatment ends →	Every 6 to 12 months, or as needed • Physical exam • CBC with differential
Procedures and molecular testing	Bone marrow aspirate is possible as often as 3 to 6 months for at least 5 years • If bone marrow aspirate is done: Flow cytometry with additional studies that may include cytogenetics, FISH, molecular testing, and MRD testing.	
	Periodic *BCR-ABL1* testing if Ph+ ALL	

Relapse

When leukemia returns after a period of remission, it is called a relapse. The goal of treatment is to achieve remission again. A relapse is very serious. It is important to ask about prognosis.

Those with relapsed ALL are placed into risk groups. Length of first complete remission (CR1) and site of relapse are two important factors. Relapse can occur in the bone marrow called isolated medullary relapse, in areas outside of the marrow or blood such the brain or testicles called isolated extramedullary relapse, or a combination of both. In general, those with a later relapse, 3 or more years after starting treatment, have the best prognosis.

Refractory

When leukemia remains and does not respond to treatment, it is called refractory or resistant cancer. The cancer may be resistant at the start of treatment or it may become resistant during treatment. Refractory disease is very serious. It is important to ask about prognosis.

Review

- The goal of treatment is a complete response.
- Induction is the first stage of treatment. You will likely spend time in the hospital for part of this treatment.
- Consolidation or post-induction therapy is the second stage of treatment. It is needed to kill any cancer cells called minimal or measurable residual disease (MRD) that might be left after induction. Consolidation usually lasts 6 to 9 months.
- Maintenance or post-consolidation therapy is the final phase of treatment. It usually lasts 2 years.
- Central nervous system (CNS) prophylaxis is given to prevent ALL from spreading to the brain and spinal fluid.
- Monitoring watches for any changes in your condition.
- ALL that returns after remission is called relapse. To prevent relapse, it is important to take your medicine as prescribed and not miss or skip any doses.
- When ALL does not respond to treatment or stops responding to treatment, it is called refractory or resistant cancer.

4

Treating ALL

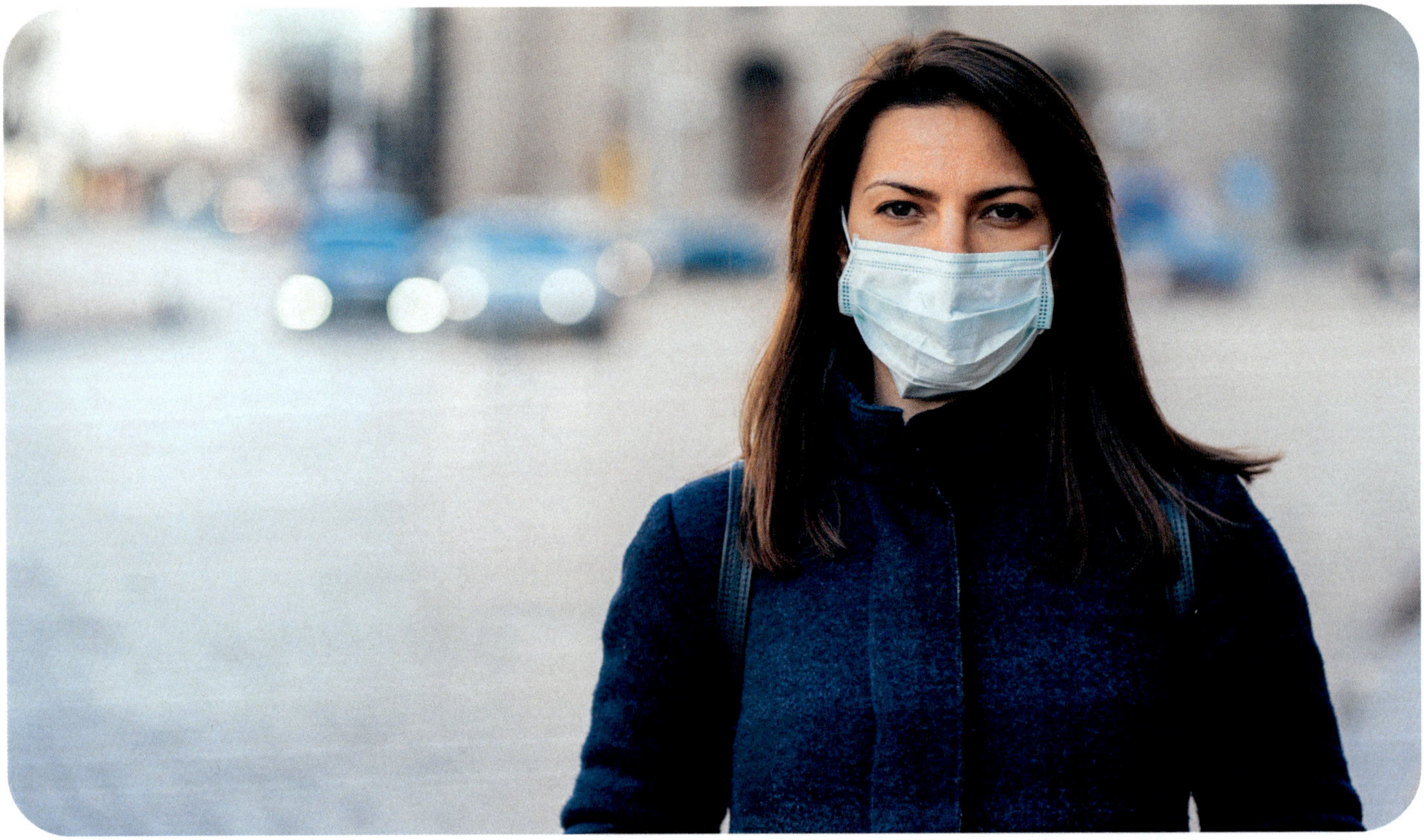

There is more than one treatment for ALL. This chapter presents an overview of the possible types of treatment and what to expect. Not everyone will receive the same treatment. Treatment options are based on many factors. Together, you and your doctor will choose a treatment plan that is right for you.

Overview

Chemotherapy is the backbone of ALL treatment and is often combined with other drug therapies. Chemotherapy is a type of systemic drug therapy that kills fast-growing cells throughout the body, including cancer cells and normal cells.

Chemotherapy, fluids, and blood products might be given through:

- Central venous access device (CVAD)
- Peripheral intravenous line (PIV)

You will likely get either a catheter or a port to deliver chemotherapy and other treatments. A catheter is a thin, long tube that is often placed in the chest. This goes into a large vein and stays there until treatment is complete. A port is a small, round disc that is usually placed in the chest.

CVAD

A central venous access device (CVAD) and central venous catheter (CVC or central line) are devices inserted into the body through a vein. This makes it easier to give fluids, blood products, medicine, and other therapies directly into the bloodstream. The device may be a catheter (examples include Hickman and Broviac) or port (port-a-cath). The device will be inserted during a minor surgery and remain in your body until treatment is complete. Once the CVAD is removed, the skin will heal.

CVADs can be inserted into a vein in the neck (jugular) or under the collarbone (subclavian). It can be inserted into one of the peripheral veins of the upper arm. While generally safe, there are risks for infection and blood clots.

PICC

A peripherally inserted central catheter (PICC or PICC line) is a long, thin tube that's inserted through a vein in your arm and passed through to the larger veins near your heart.

PIV

A peripheral intravenous line (PIV) is a small, short plastic catheter that is placed through the skin into a vein, usually in the hand, elbow, or foot. A PIV can be used to give fluids, medicines, and certain chemotherapies.

Chemotherapy

Chemotherapy can be given as follows:

- **Oral (PO)** – taken by mouth either as a liquid or pill
- **Subcutaneous (SQ)** – given under the skin
- **Intramuscular (IM)** – uses a needle to inject medicine in the muscle of the arm or leg (like the flu shot)
- **IV (intravenous) infusion** – chemotherapy administered through a vein using IV push, gravity infusion, or infusion pump. In an IV push, a drug is injected quickly over a few minutes. With a gravity infusion, medicine is put into a bag that hangs on a pole, and the pressure of gravity delivers the medicine into the IV line at a safe and steady rate. In an IV infusion, chemotherapy flows through a tube attached to the catheter. The flow may be controlled by a machine called an IV pump.
- **Intrathecal (IT)** – chemotherapy administered into the spinal fluid. In addition to other forms of chemotherapy, you will have chemotherapy injected into the cerebrospinal fluid (CSF) to kill any leukemia cells that might have spread to the brain and spinal cord. This treatment is given through a lumbar puncture (spinal tap).

Types of chemotherapy

Chemotherapies used to treat ALL disrupt the life cycle of cancer cells. There are many types of chemotherapy used to treat ALL. Often chemotherapies are combined. This is called multiagent chemotherapy.

Some types of chemotherapies used to treat ALL are described next.

Alkylating agents

Alkylating agents damage DNA by adding a chemical to it. This group of drugs includes cyclophosphamide.

Anthracyclines

Anthracyclines damage and disrupt the making of DNA causing cell death of both cancerous and non-cancerous cells.

Examples of anthracyclines include:

- Daunorubicin (Cerubidine®)
- Idarubicin (Idamycin PFS®)
- Doxorubicin (adriamycin)

Antimetabolites

Antimetabolites prevent the “building blocks” of DNA from being used.

Examples of antimetabolites include:

- Cytarabine (Cytosar-U®)
- Fludarabine (Fludara®)
- Clofarabine (Clolar®)
- Methotrexate
- 6-MP (6-mercaptopurine)
- Nelarabine (Arranon®)

Did you know?

The terms "chemotherapy" and "systemic therapy" are often used interchangeably, but they are not the same. Chemotherapy, targeted therapy, and immunotherapy are all types of systemic therapy.

Enzyme therapy

All cells in the body need the amino acid asparagine to survive. Normal white blood cells can make their own asparagine, but cancerous white blood cells cannot. Asparaginase is an enzyme that speeds up the breakdown of asparagine in the blood. This lowers the level of asparagine in the body. Without asparagine, leukemia cells die.

Pegaspargase (Oncaspar®), calaspargase (Asparlas™), or asparaginase derived from *Erwinia chrysanthemi* (Erwinaze® or ERW) are some types of enzyme therapy used in chemotherapy treatment.

Plant alkaloids

Plant alkaloids are made from plants. Plant alkaloids are cell-cycle specific. This means they attack the cells during various phases of division. Vincristine (also known as Oncovin® or Vincasar PFS®) belongs in a class of drugs called vinca alkaloids. It is also a microtubule inhibitor. Microtubule inhibitors stop a cell from dividing into two cells.

Steroids

Steroid is the short name for corticosteroid. Steroids are man-made versions of hormones made by the adrenal glands. The adrenal glands are small structures found near the kidneys, which help regulate blood pressure and reduce inflammation.

Steroids also are toxic to lymphoid cells and are an important part of ALL chemotherapy. Steroids can cause short-term and long-term side effects. Corticosteroids are not the same as the steroids used by some athletes.

Steroids include:

- Dexamethasone
- Prednisone
- Hydrocortisone

Targeted therapy

Targeted therapy is a form of systemic therapy that works throughout your body. It is a drug therapy that focuses on specific or unique features of cancer cells.

Targeted therapies seek out how cancer cells grow, divide, and move in the body. These drugs stop the action of molecules that help cancer cells grow and/or survive.

Tyrosine kinase inhibitor

A tyrosine kinase inhibitor (TKI) is a type of targeted therapy that blocks the signals that cause cancer to grow and spread. TKIs might be used alone or in combination with other systemic therapies like chemotherapy.

Tyrosine kinases are proteins in cells that are important for many cell functions. The protein made by the *BCR-ABL1* gene is a tyrosine kinase. It moves or transfers chemicals, called phosphates, from one molecule to another. TKIs block this transfer, which stops cell growth.

Each TKI works in a slightly different way. You might not be given a certain TKI if you have a health condition, such as lung or heart issues, or certain mutations. Sometimes, a TKI will stop working when there's a new mutation in ALL cells. Switching to a different TKI may help.

TKIs used to treat ALL

TKIs that might be used to treat ALL:

- Bosutinib (Bosulif®)
- Dasatinib (Sprycel®)
- Imatinib (Gleevec®)
- Nilotinib (Tasigna®)
- Ponatinib (Iclusig®)

TKIs are divided into first, second, and even third generation. Each generation of drug gets more specific and better at targeting certain mutations. This means that next-generation TKIs are usually more effective and faster at creating a response. However, they might have more side effects.

Imatinib is the only first-generation TKI. Since it is less toxic than second-generation TKIs, it is a good option for those who are older or who have other more serious health issues. Risks of each TKI are considered for your specific situation.

If ALL doesn't seem to be responding to one TKI, then another TKI will be tried. Certain drugs may work better and be less toxic. Dose might be increased or decreased depending on how ALL is responding to treatment. You will be closely monitored during treatment.

Tell your doctor about any medicines, vitamins, over-the-counter drugs, herbals, or supplements you are taking.

Warnings!

You might be asked to stop taking or avoid certain herbal supplements when on a TKI, chemotherapy, or steroid. Some supplements can affect the ability of a drug to do its job. This is called a drug interaction. It is critical to speak with your care team about any supplements you may be taking.

Some examples include:

- Turmeric
- Gingko biloba
- Green tea extract
- St. John's Wort

Even certain medicines can affect the ability of a TKI to do its job. Antacids, heart medicine, and antidepressants are just some of the medicines that might interact with a targeted therapy. This is why it is important to tell your doctor about any medications, vitamins, over-the-counter (OTC) drugs, herbals, or supplements you are taking. **Bring a list with you to every visit.**

Immunotherapy

Immunotherapy is a targeted therapy that increases the activity of your immune system. By doing so, it improves your body's ability to find and destroy cancer cells. Immunotherapy can be given alone or with other types of treatment. Immunotherapies are sometimes used for relapsed/refractory disease.

Monoclonal antibody therapy

Antibody therapy uses antibodies to help the body fight cancer, infection, or other diseases. Antibodies are proteins made by the immune system that bind to specific markers on cells or tissues. Monoclonal antibodies are a type of antibody made in the lab. In cancer treatment, monoclonal antibodies may kill cancer or leukemia cells directly, they may block development of tumor blood vessels, or they may help the immune system kill cancer cells.

- Blinatumomab (Blincyto®) allows normal T cells to attack cancerous B cells by bringing them close together. It specifically targets the CD19 antigen present on B cells. Blinatumomab may cause severe, life-threatening, or fatal reactions.
- Inotuzumab ozogamicin (Besponsa™) binds to CD22 on leukemia cells then releases a toxic agent once it's inside the cells.
- Rituximab (Rituxan®) works against the protein CD20 found on the surface of B cells. When it binds to this protein it triggers cell death.

CD19-targeting CAR T-cell therapy

CD19-directed genetically modified autologous T-cell immunotherapy is made from your own T cells. T cells will be removed from your body, and in the lab, a CAR (chimeric antigen receptor) will be added to them. This programs the T cells to find leukemia cells. The programmed T cells will be infused back into your body to find and kill cancer cells. This treatment is not for everyone. There can be severe and sometimes life-threatening reactions.

Tisagenlecleucel (Kymriah™) is a type of CD19-targeting CAR T-cell therapy. It is only used in those under 26 years of age with refractory B-ALL disease or 2 or more relapses.

More information on CAR T-cell therapy can be found in *NCCN Guidelines for Patients: Immunotherapy Side Effects*, available at NCCN.org/patientguidelines.

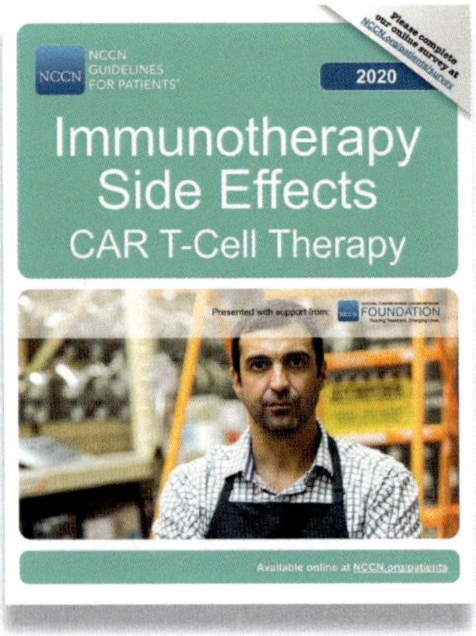

Radiation therapy

Radiation therapy (RT) uses high-energy radiation from x-rays, gamma rays, protons, and other sources to kill cancer cells and shrink tumors. It is given over a certain period of time. Radiation therapy can be given alone or with certain systemic therapies. It may be used as supportive care to help ease pain or discomfort caused by cancer.

- Those with leukemia in the central nervous system at diagnosis may receive radiation to the brain area.
- Those with testicular disease at diagnosis that remains after induction therapy may receive radiation to the testes.

Cranial irradiation

In cranial irradiation, the areas of the brain targeted for ALL radiation treatment are different from areas targeted for brain metastases of solid tumors. Cranial irradiation might be given to prevent ALL from spreading to the brain. This is called prophylaxis.

Total body irradiation

Total body irradiation (TBI) is radiation of the whole body given before bone marrow transplant.

Stem cell transplant

A stem cell transplant (SCT) replaces bone marrow stem cells. You might hear it called a hematopoietic cell transplant (HCT). This book will refer to it as SCT.

There are 2 types of SCTs:

- Autologous – stem cells come from you
- Allogeneic – stem cells come from a donor who may or may not be related to you

Only an allogeneic SCT (allo-SCT) is used as a treatment option for ALL. An SCT depends upon donor availability and your health at the time of potential SCT. The steps of an allogeneic SCT are described next.

Conditioning

Before an SCT, treatment is needed to destroy bone marrow cells. This is called conditioning and it creates room for the healthy donor stem cells. It also weakens the immune system so your body won't kill the transplanted cells.

Chemotherapy is used for conditioning. Radiation therapy may also be given as part of conditioning treatment.

Transplanting stem cells

After conditioning, you will receive the healthy stem cells through a transfusion. A transfusion is a slow injection of blood products into a vein. This can take several hours. The transplanted stem cells will travel to your bone marrow and grow. New, healthy blood cells will form. This is called engraftment. It usually takes about 2 to 4 weeks.

Until then, you will have little or no immune defense. You may need to stay in a very clean room at the hospital or be given antibiotics to prevent or treat infection. Transfusions are also possible. A red blood cell transfusion is used to prevent bleeding and to treat anemia (below normal red blood cell count). A platelet transfusion is used to treat a low platelet count or bleeding. While waiting for the cells to engraft, you will likely feel tired and weak.

Possible side effects

Every treatment has side effects. You will be monitored for infections, disease relapse, and graft-versus-host disease (GVHD). In GVHD, the donor cells attack your normal, healthy tissue. There are treatments for GVHD. Ask about the possible side effects or complications of SCT and how this might affect your quality of life.

Clinical trials

A clinical trial is a type of medical research study. After being developed and tested in a laboratory, potential new ways of fighting cancer need to be studied in people. If found to be safe and effective in a clinical trial, a drug, device, or treatment approach may be approved by the U.S. Food and Drug Administration (FDA). Everyone with cancer should carefully consider all of the treatment options available for their cancer type, including standard treatments and clinical trials. Talk to your treatment team about whether a clinical trial might make sense for you.

Phases

Most cancer clinical trials focus on treatment. Treatment trials are done in phases that build on one another.

- Phase I trials study the safety and side effects of an investigational drug or treatment approach.
- Phase II trials study how well the drug or approach works against a specific type of cancer.
- Phase III trials test the drug or approach against a standard treatment. If the results are good, it may be approved by the FDA.
- Phase IV trials study the long-term safety and benefit of an FDA-approved treatment.

Who can enroll?

Every clinical trial has rules for joining, called eligibility criteria. The rules may be about age, cancer type and stage, treatment history, or general health. These requirements ensure that participants are alike in specific ways and that the treatment is as safe as possible.

Informed consent

Clinical trials are managed by a group of experts called a research team. The research team will review the study with you in detail, including its purpose and the risks and benefits of joining. This information is also described in detail in an informed consent form. Giving informed consent means that you understand the possible benefits and risks and agree to join. Read the form carefully and ask questions before signing it. Take time to discuss with family, friends, or others you trust. Keep in mind that you can leave and seek treatment outside of the clinical trial at any time.

Start the conversation

Don't wait for your doctor to bring up clinical trials. Start the conversation and learn about all of your treatment options. If you find a study that you may be eligible for, ask your treatment team if you meet the requirements. Try not to be discouraged if you cannot join. New clinical trials are always becoming available.

Frequently asked questions

There are many myths and misconceptions surrounding clinical trials. The possible benefits and risks are not well understood by many with cancer.

What if I get the placebo?

A placebo is an inactive version of a real medicine. Placebos are almost never used alone in cancer clinical trials. All participants receive cancer treatment. You may receive a commonly used treatment, the investigational drug, or both.

Do I have to pay to be in a clinical trial?

Rarely. It depends on the study, your health insurance, and the state in which you live. Your treatment team and the research team can help determine if you are responsible for any costs.

Supportive care

Supportive care will be specific to your needs. Supportive care is health care that relieves symptoms caused by cancer or its treatment and improves quality of life. It might include pain relief (palliative care), emotional or spiritual support, financial aid, or family counseling. Supportive care and palliative care are often used interchangeably. Supportive care is always given.

Some potential side effects and procedures are described next. They are not listed in order of importance. Some side effects are very rare.

Side effects

All cancer treatments can cause unwanted health issues called side effects. Side effects depend on many factors. These factors include the drug type and dose, length of treatment, and the person. Some side effects may be harmful to your health. Others may just be unpleasant. ALL treatment can cause a number of side effects. Some are very serious.

Late effects

Late effects are side effects that occur months or years after a disease is diagnosed or after treatment has ended. Late effects may be caused by cancer or cancer treatment. They may include physical, mental, and social problems, and second cancers. The sooner late effects are treated the better. Ask your care team about what late effects could occur. This will help you know what to look for.

Blood clots

Cancer treatment can cause blood clots to form. This can block blood flow and oxygen in the body. Blood clots can break loose and travel to other parts of the body causing stroke or other problems.

Cytokine release syndrome

Cytokine release syndrome (CRS) is a condition that may occur after treatment with some types of immunotherapy, such as monoclonal antibodies and CAR T cells. It is caused by a large, rapid release of cytokines from immune cells affected by the immunotherapy. Signs and symptoms of CRS include fever, muscle aches, nausea, headache, rash, fast heartbeat, low blood pressure, and trouble breathing.

Dialysis

There are different types of dialysis. Dialysis is the process of filtering blood when the kidneys are unable. Hemodialysis and hemofiltration remove waste and water by circulating blood outside the body through an external filter. Dialysis is uncommon in ALL.

Distress

Distress is an unpleasant experience of a mental, physical, social, or spiritual nature. It can affect how you feel, think, and act. Distress might include feelings of sadness, fear, helplessness, worry, anger, and guilt. You may also experience depression, anxiety, and sleeping problems.

For more information, read *NCCN Guidelines for Patients: Distress During Cancer Care,* available at NCCN.org/patientguidelines.

High blood pressure

High blood pressure (HBP or hypertension) occurs when the force of blood flowing through your blood vessels is consistently too high. This can cause headaches and vision problems. If left untreated, HPB can cause heart problems and stroke. Steroids can cause HBP. Medicine might be used to control HBP.

High blood sugar

One possible side effect of steroids is high blood sugar or hyperglycemia. Glucose (sugar found in the blood) will be measured. Insulin might be needed to control high blood sugar.

Hyperleukocytosis

Hyperleukocytosis (leukostasis) is an extremely high lymphoblast count.

Hypersensitivity, allergy, and anaphylaxis

Certain treatments can cause an unwanted reaction. Hypersensitivity is an exaggerated response by the immune system to a drug or other substance. This can include hives, skin welts, and trouble breathing. An allergy is an immune reaction to a substance that normally is harmless or would not cause an immune response in most people. An allergic response may cause harmful symptoms such as itching or inflammation (swelling). Anaphylaxis or anaphylactic shock is a severe and possible life-threatening allergic reaction.

Infection

You will be monitored for signs of infection. Fever can be a sign of infection. People are at a higher risk for infection when they have neutropenia. Neutropenia is an abnormally low number of neutrophils (a type of white blood cell) in the blood. Neutrophils make up nearly half of all white blood cells and are the first line of defense when infection strikes. Antibiotics might be used to treat infection. Blood or urine may be tested when infection is suspected.

For more information, read the *NCCN Guidelines for Patients: Anemia and Neutropenia,* available at NCCN.org/patientguidelines.

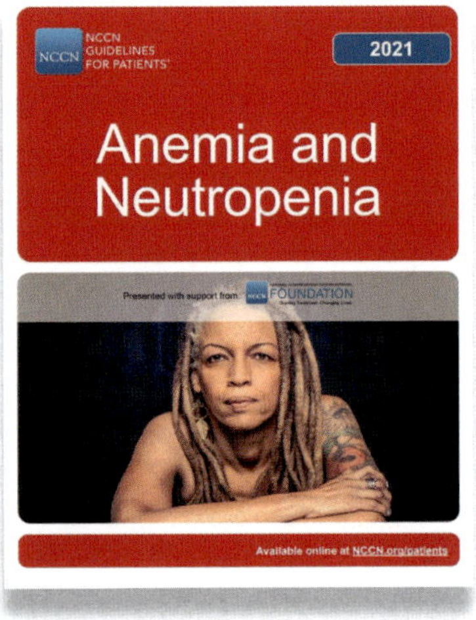

Leukapheresis

In leukapheresis, you will be connected to a machine called a centrifuge. The centrifuge separates white blood cells (leukocytes) from other blood cells. Once the excess leukocytes are removed, the blood is returned to your body. It is also called leukocytapheresis.

Nausea and vomiting

Nausea and vomiting are a common side effect of treatment. You will be given medicine to prevent nausea and vomiting.

For more information, read the *NCCN Guidelines for Patients: Nausea and Vomiting*, available at NCCN.org/patientguidelines.

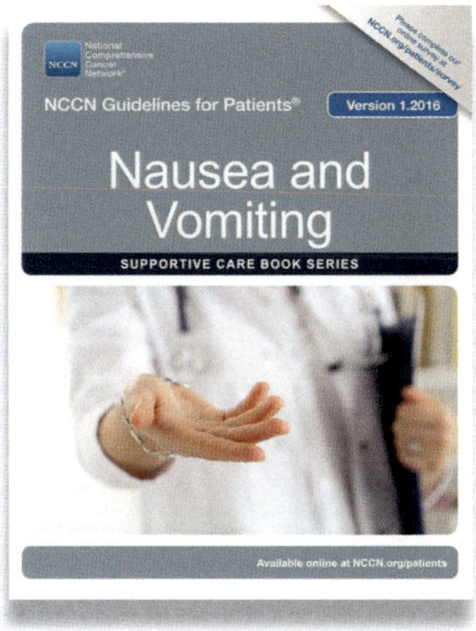

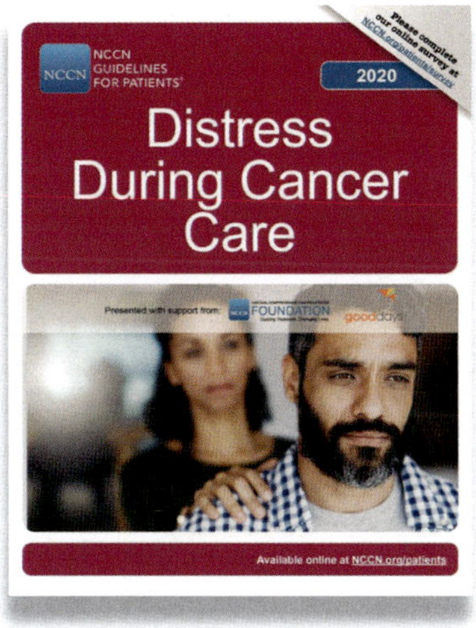

Neurocognitive effects

Some treatments can damage the nervous system (neurotoxicity) causing problems with concentration and memory. Survivors are at risk for neurotoxicity and might be recommended for neuropsychological testing. Neuropsychology looks at how the health of your brain affects your thinking and behavior. Neuropsychological testing can identify your limits and doctors can create a plan to help with these limits.

Neurotoxicity

If ALL treatment includes methotrexate, then you will be monitored for methotrexate neurotoxicity (MTX). Neurotoxicity, such as seizures and confusion, can be seen with immunotherapy, as well.

Finding a clinical trial

In the Unites States

NCCN Cancer Centers
NCCN.org/cancercenters

The National Cancer Institute (NCI)
cancer.gov/about-cancer/treatment/clinical-trials/search

Worldwide

The U.S. National Library of Medicine (NLM)
clinicaltrials.gov/

Help finding a clinical trial
is available from
NCI's Cancer Information Service (CIS)
1.800.4.CANCER (1.800.422.6237)
cancer.gov/contact

Neuropathy

Neuropathy is a nerve problem that causes pain, numbness, tingling, swelling, or muscle weakness in different parts of the body. It usually begins in the hands or feet and gets worse over time. Neuropathy may be caused by cancer or cancer treatment such as vincristine.

Organ issues

Treatment might cause your kidneys, liver, heart, and pancreas to not to work as well as they should.

Osteonecrosis

Osteonecrosis, or avascular necrosis, is death of bone tissue due to lack of blood supply. It is a possible side effect of steroids and most often affects weight-bearing joints, such as the hip and/or knee.

Pain

Tell your care team about any pain or discomfort. You might meet with a palliative care specialist to manage pain. Bone pain and vincristine-associated neuropathic pain are common in ALL.

Pneumonia

Pneumocystis pneumonia is a serious infection caused by the fungus *Pneumocystis jirovecii*. Since those with ALL are at high risk, medicine will be given throughout treatment to prevent this type of pneumonia.

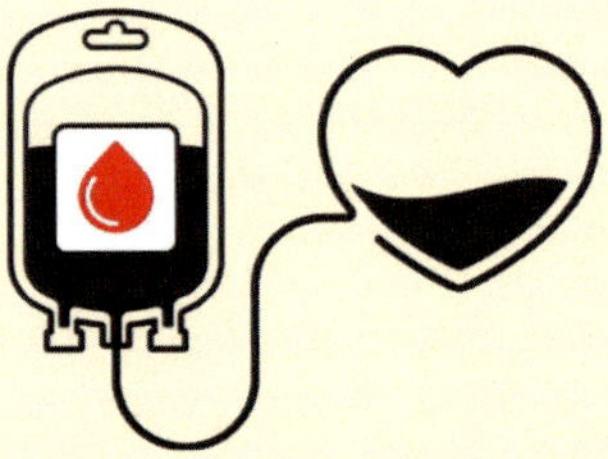

Transfusions

A transfusion is a common procedure to replace blood or blood components (red blood cells or platelets). It is given to you through an intravenous line (IV), a tiny tube that is inserted into a vein with a small needle.

- The whole process can take about 1 to 4 hours, depending on how much blood is needed.
- Most transfusions use blood from a donor. Some people choose a family member or friend to donate blood.
- Blood transfusions are usually very safe. Donated blood is carefully tested, handled, and stored.
- Most people's bodies handle blood transfusions very well. But, like any medical procedure, there are some risks. Speak with your doctor for specific information about your risks.
- Chemotherapy can affect how bone marrow makes new blood cells. Some people getting treatment for cancer might need a transfusion of red blood cells or platelets.

Survivorship

A survivor is someone with a history of cancer. A person is a cancer survivor from the time of diagnosis until end of life. When treatment leads to remission (or no evidence of disease), you will need follow-up or survivorship care. Seek out peer support groups, whether online or in-person.

For more information, see NCCN.org/patientguidelines.

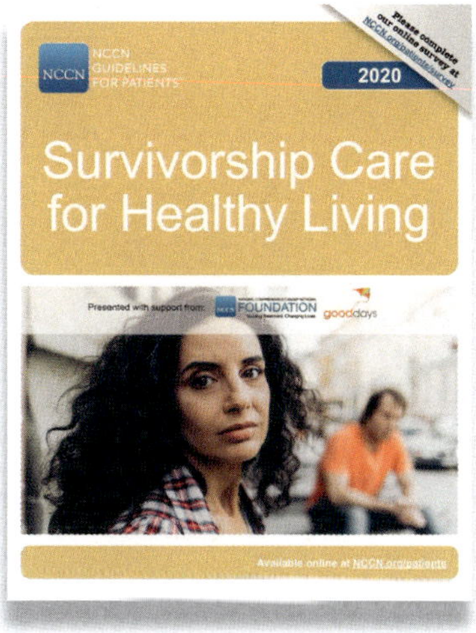

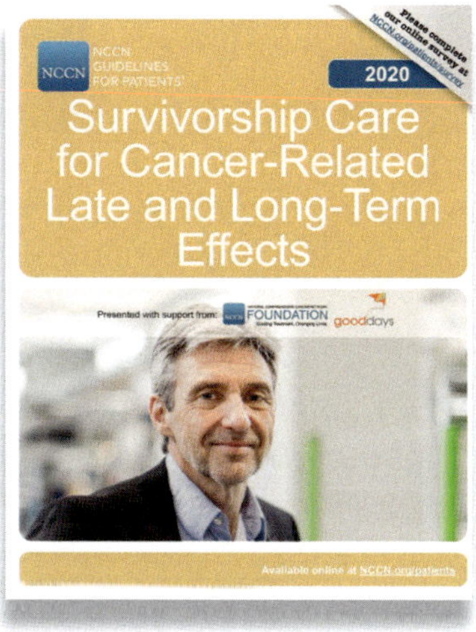

Therapy-related toxicity

Many of the drug therapies used to treat ALL can be harmful to the body. You will be closely monitored for therapy-related toxicity.

Transfusions

Blood transfusions are common during ALL treatment. A transfusion is a slow injection of blood products such as red blood cells or platelets into a vein. Over time, the body may begin to reject blood transfusions.

Trouble eating

Sometimes side effects from surgery, cancer, or its treatment might cause you to feel not hungry or sick to your stomach (nauseated). You might have a sore mouth. Healthy eating is important during treatment. It includes eating a balanced diet, eating the right amount of food, and drinking enough fluids. A registered dietitian who is an expert in nutrition and food can help. Speak to your care team if you have trouble eating or maintaining weight.

Tumor lysis syndrome

Tumor lysis syndrome (TLS) causes an imbalance of substances in blood. There are different treatments for TLS. Treatment depends on what substances are out of balance and how well your kidneys are working. Sometimes, TLS can cause too much potassium in your blood. Treatment might include hemodialysis or hemofiltration. A machine will filter your blood.

Weight gain

Weight gain is one side effect of high-dose steroids. This can be uncomfortable and cause distress. It is important to maintain muscle mass. Try to find an activity you enjoy. Ask your care team what can be done to help manage weight gain.

Review

- Chemotherapy kills fast-growing cells throughout the body, including cancer cells and normal cells.
- Steroids are part of ALL regimens.
- Targeted therapy focuses on specific or unique features of cancer cells.
- Immunotherapy increases the activity of your immune system.
- A stem cell transplant (SCT) replaces damaged bone marrow stem cells with healthy stem cells. You might hear it called a hematopoietic cell transplant (HCT) or bone marrow transplant (BMT).
- Clinical trials study how safe and helpful tests and treatments are for people. Many ALL treatment regimens are the result of clinical trials.
- Supportive care is health care that relieves symptoms caused by cancer or its treatment and improves quality of life. Supportive care is always given.
- All cancer treatments can cause unwanted health issues called side effects. You will be monitored for side effects, infection, and other treatment-related issues.
- Some side effects, called late effects, may take years to appear. Risk for late effects will depend on the type(s) of cancer treatment you had, and the dose and the length of time you were treated. It is important to go to follow-up appointments.

Get to know your care team and let them get to know you.

5 Ph+ B-ALL

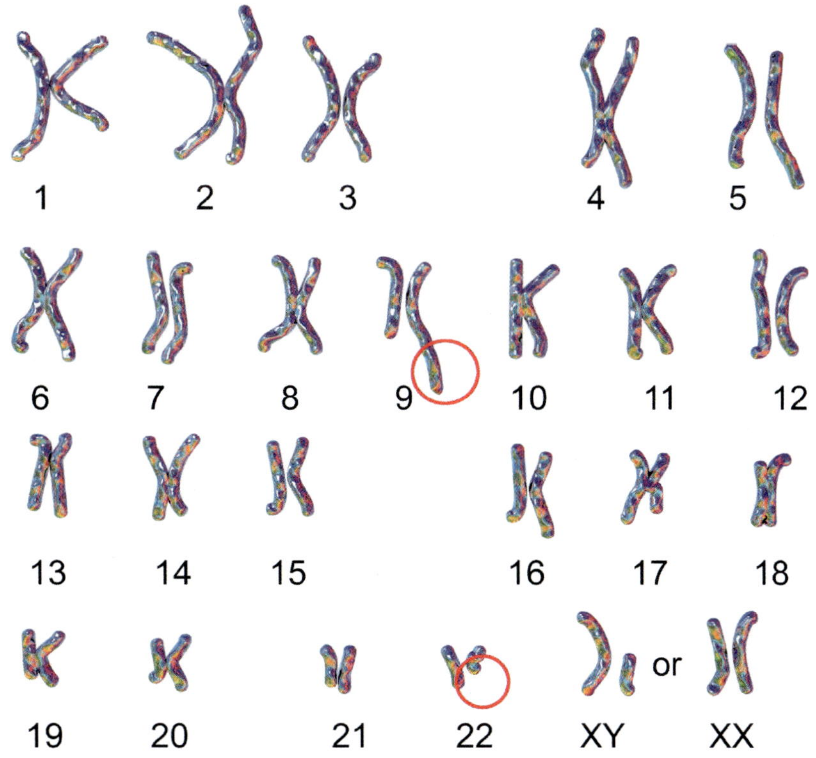

In Ph-positive (Ph+) B-ALL, tests show the presence of the Philadelphia chromosome. This happens when a piece of chromosome 9 and a piece of chromosome 22 break off and trade places with each other. The result is a fused gene called *BCR-ABL1*. Treatment is usually an intensive combination of systemic therapies.

Overview

Ph+ B-ALL is less common than other types of B-ALL. Treatment aims to stop the activity of the BCR-ABL fusion protein. Although Ph+ B-ALL is considered high risk, there are effective treatments such as imatinib, a tyrosine kinase inhibitor (TKI) that targets the BCR-ABL fusion protein, and other TKIs such as dasatinib, nilotinib, bosutinib, and ponatinib. Treatment is usually an intensive combination of systemic therapies. Systemic therapies work throughout the body.

Age and health

Age or serious health issues may impact treatment. AYAs and adults under 65 years of age who do not have other serious health conditions can tolerate higher-dose or more intense treatment regimens.

Adults who are 65 years of age and over or those who have serious health conditions may have modified treatment regimens. Age is just a guideline. Your overall health and fitness play a role. Depending on your health and other factors, you might receive a lower-dose treatment. This does not mean it is less effective.

Induction

There are 3 induction options:

- Clinical trial
- TKI with chemotherapy
- TKI with steroid

There are a many TKIs and chemotherapies used to treat ALL. Talk with your doctor about which treatment might be best for you. All regimens include central nervous system (CNS) prophylaxis with systemic therapy and/or intrathecal (IT) therapy. This is treatment to prevent CNS disease.

Treatment response will be measured after completing induction. The goal is a complete response (CR). In less than a CR, cancer remains. Treatment will follow relapsed or refractory section.

After a CR, tests will look for minimal residual disease (MRD). When MRD is found, it is called MRD-positive (MRD+).

Consolidation

Consolidation treatment is based on if any minimal residual disease is found. For consolidation treatment options following a complete response (CR), see Guide 5.

MRD+

Persistent or rising MRD is treated with:

- Blinatumomab with or without TKI (if B-ALL) or
- You might continue with multiagent chemotherapy with steroid and TKI or
- An allogeneic stem cell transplant (allo-SCT)

After consolidation, an allo-SCT might be an option. An SCT depends upon donor availability and your health at the time of potential SCT. An SCT is not an option for everyone. You might be given a TKI after an allo-SCT.

MRD-

If MRD is negative (MRD-), then you will continue multiagent chemotherapy with steroid and TKI. If MRD remains negative after consolidation, then maintenance therapy with a TKI will be given.

Surveillance and monitoring

During maintenance or after a stem cell transplant, you will be monitored for signs of recurrence called relapse.

Guide 5
Consolidation options after a complete response (CR)

MRD+ (persistent or rising MRD)	Blinatumomab with or without TKI (for B-ALL)	→ Allo-SCT (might be followed with TKI)
	Continue multiagent chemotherapy with steroid and TKI	→ Allo-SCT (might be followed with TKI)
	Allo-SCT, in some cases (might be followed by TKI)	
MRD-	Continue multiagent chemotherapy with steroid and TKI followed by maintenance therapy with TKI	
	Allo-SCT, in some cases (might be followed by TKI)	

Relapsed or refractory disease

Relapse is the return of cancer after a period of remission. The goal of treatment is to achieve remission again. Cancer can return in the bone marrow called isolated medullary relapse, outside the bone marrow called isolated extramedullary relapse, or a combination of both (combined relapse). Extramedullary relapse can occur in the central nervous system or testicles. Location of relapse will impact treatment.

Relapse can happen more than once. With each relapse the goal of treatment is a complete response or remission. When cancer returns only in the bone marrow, it is called isolated medullary relapse. When cancer is found in the central nervous system and testicles, but not in the bone marrow or blood, it is called isolated extramedullary relapse. In this case, systemic therapy is needed to prevent relapse in bone marrow.

When leukemia remains and does not respond to treatment, it is called refractory.

Before starting treatment for relapsed or refractory disease, you will have *ABL1* kinase domain mutation testing. For treatment options, see Guide 6.

Treatment options for relapsed or refractory disease include:

- Clinical trial
- TKI with or without chemotherapy
- TKI with or without steroid
- Blinatumomab with or without TKI
- Inotuzumab ozogamicin with or without bosutinib (TKI intolerant or refractory B-ALL)
- Tisagenlecleucel

Tisagenlecleucel is an option in those under 26 years of age with refractory B-ALL disease or in those who have had 2 or more relapses and failure of 2 TKIs.

Treatment response will be checked. Next step would be an SCT.

Guide 6
Relapse or refractory disease: Ph+ B-ALL

Treatment options	• Clinical trial • TKI with or without chemotherapy • TKI with or without steroid • Blinatumomab with or without TKI • Inotuzumab ozogamicin with or without bosutinib (TKI intolerant or refractory B-ALL) • Tisagenlecleucel (in those under 26 years of age with refractory B-ALL disease or 2 or more relapses)	→	Consider an allo-SCT

Review

- In Ph-positive (Ph+) B-ALL, tests show the presence of the Philadelphia chromosome.
- Induction is either a clinical trial or systemic therapy.
- All treatment regimens include systemic and/or intrathecal (IT) therapy to prevent central nervous system (CNS) disease.
- Treatment response will be measured after completing induction. The goal is a complete response (CR).
- After a CR, tests will look for minimal residual disease (MRD). When MRD is found, it is called MRD-positive (MRD+).
- Treatment for MRD+ aims to reduce the amount of MRD.
- During maintenance or after a stem cell transplant, you will be monitored for signs of recurrence called relapse.
- Relapse can happen more than once. With each relapse the goal of treatment is a complete response or remission.
- An SCT depends upon donor availability and your health at the time of potential SCT.

An important note about teens

✓ Teens are less likely to take their medicine. Help your teen feel in control by finding a routine that works for them.

✓ Talk to your teen about how to refill prescriptions and what to do so they don't run out of medicine.

6

Ph- B-ALL

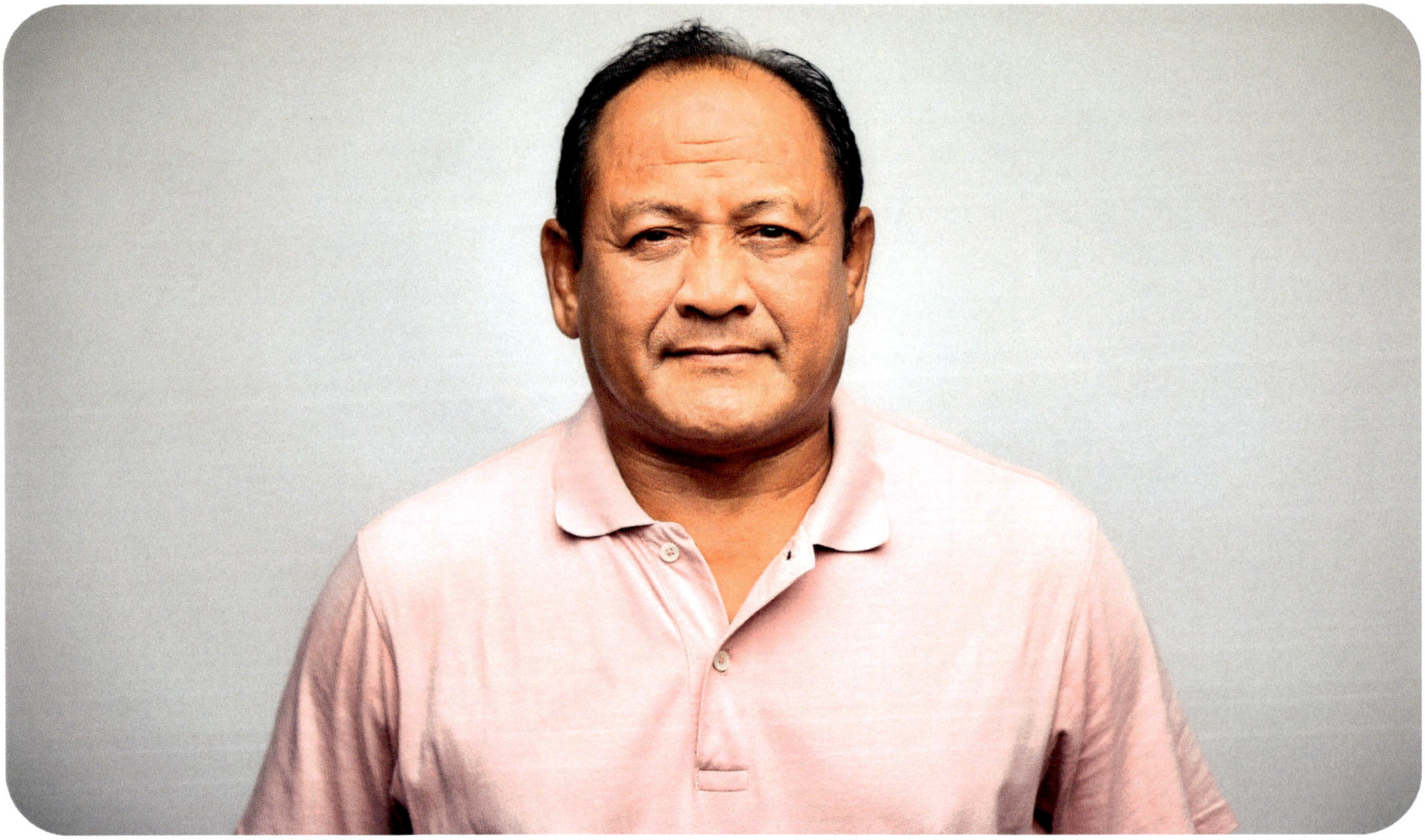

Philadelphia chromosome-negative (Ph-) B-ALL is the most common type of B-ALL. Treatment is a clinical trial or systemic therapy.

Overview

Ph-negative (Ph-) does not have the Philadelphia chromosome. It is the most common type of B-ALL. Induction will either be a clinical trial or multiagent chemotherapy. All regimens include central nervous system (CNS) prophylaxis with systemic therapy and/or intrathecal (IT) therapy. Treatment response will be measured after completing induction. Consolidation is based on if tests find minimal residual disease (MRD).

Age and health

Age or serious health issues may impact treatment. AYAs and adults under 65 years of age who do not have other serious health conditions can tolerate higher-dose or more intense treatment regimens.

Adults who are 65 years of age and over or those who have serious health conditions may have modified treatment regimens. Age is just a guideline. Your overall health and fitness play a role. Depending on your health and other factors, you might receive a lower-dose treatment. This does not mean it is less effective.

Induction

Induction options include:

- Clinical trial
- Multiagent chemotherapy

Adults who are 65 years of age and over or those who have serious health conditions may opt for a palliative steroid instead of a clinical trial or chemotherapy. For AYAs, a pediatric-based treatment regimen is preferred.

Many induction treatment regimens are part of ongoing clinical trials. Induction is a combination of systemic therapies. Systemic therapies work throughout the body. All treatment regimens include systemic and/or intrathecal therapy (injected into the spinal fluid) to prevent CNS disease. This is treatment to prevent CNS disease.

Treatment response will be measured after completing induction. The goal is a complete response (CR). After a complete response, you will be monitored for minimal residual disease (MRD). When MRD is found, it is called MRD-positive (MRD+). In less than a CR, cancer remains. Treatment will follow relapsed or refractory section.

Consolidation

Consolidation options are based on if tests find minimal residual disease. See Guide 7.

MRD+

In general, MRD positivity at the end of induction predicts a high chance of relapse. Treatment is usually an allogeneic stem cell transplant (allo-SCT). Therapy aimed at eliminating MRD prior to an allo-SCT is preferred, when possible. For B-ALL, you might be given blinatumomab before an allo-SCT.

MRD-

If no minimal residual disease is found, then you will continue chemotherapy followed by maintenance therapy. An allo-SCT is also an option.

MRD unavailable

If MRD cannot be determined, then an allo-SCT is an option. You could also continue chemotherapy followed by maintenance therapy.

Allo-SCT

An allo-SCT depends upon donor availability, length of remission, your social support, and your health at the time of potential SCT.

Maintenance

Maintenance therapy is given after consolidation with multiagent chemotherapy. Maintenance is given to prevent the return or spread of ALL. It is usually a continuation of treatment, but might be at a lower dose.

Surveillance

During maintenance or after a stem cell transplant, you will be monitored for signs of recurrence.

Guide 7
Consolidation options after a complete response (CR)

MRD+	Blinatumomab (for B-ALL) followed by an allo-SCT
	Allo-SCT followed by surveillance
MRD-	Continue multiagent chemotherapy followed by maintenance therapy
	Allo-SCT followed by surveillance
MRD unavailable	Allo-SCT followed by surveillance
	Continue multiagent chemotherapy followed by maintenance therapy

Relapsed or refractory disease

Relapse is the return of cancer after a period of remission. The goal of treatment is to achieve remission again. Cancer can return in the bone marrow called isolated medullary relapse, outside the bone marrow called isolated extramedullary relapse, or a combination of both (combined relapse). Extramedullary relapse can occur in the central nervous system or testicles.

When leukemia remains and does not respond to treatment, it is called refractory.

Mutation testing and MRD assessment will be done before starting treatment. Treatment options are found in Guide 8.

Treatment options include:

- Clinical trial
- Blinatumomab
- Tisagenlecleucel - For those under 26 years of age with refractory B-ALL disease or 2 or more relapses
- Inotuzumab ozogamicin
- Chemotherapy - For those in late relapse (more than 3 years from initial diagnosis), consider treatment with the same induction regimen

Most treatment paths lead toward a stem cell transplant (SCT). The goal is to achieve an MRD-negative result before an SCT. An SCT depends upon donor availability and your health at the time of potential SCT.

Guide 8
Relapsed or refractory disease: Ph- B-ALL

Treatment options	• Clinical trial • Blinatumomab • Inotuzumab ozogamicin • Tisagenlecleucel (in those under 26 years of age with refractory B-ALL disease or 2 or more relapses) • Chemotherapy	→ Consider an allo-SCT

Multiple relapse

B-ALL can relapse multiple times. With each relapse the goal of treatment is a complete response (CR). This is not always possible.

Refractory

When leukemia remains and does not respond to treatment, it is called refractory or resistant. The cancer may be resistant at the start of treatment or it may become resistant during treatment. Refractory disease is very serious. It is important to ask about prognosis. Treatment options are the same as for relapse.

Review

- Ph-negative (Ph-) does not have the Philadelphia chromosome. It is the most common type of B-ALL.
- The goal of treatment is a complete response and to prevent the spread of cancer to areas outside the blood.
- Treatment is usually an intensive combination of systemic therapies. All regimens include central nervous system (CNS) prophylaxis with systemic therapy and/or intrathecal (IT) therapy.
- Relapse is the return of cancer after a period of remission. The goal of treatment is to achieve remission (a complete response) again.
- Cancer may be resistant at the start of treatment or it may become resistant during treatment. This is called refractory.
- For multiple relapse or refractory disease, the goal is to achieve an MRD-negative result before a stem cell transplant (SCT). An SCT is not an option for everyone.
- An SCT depends upon donor availability and your health at the time of potential SCT.

7 T-ALL

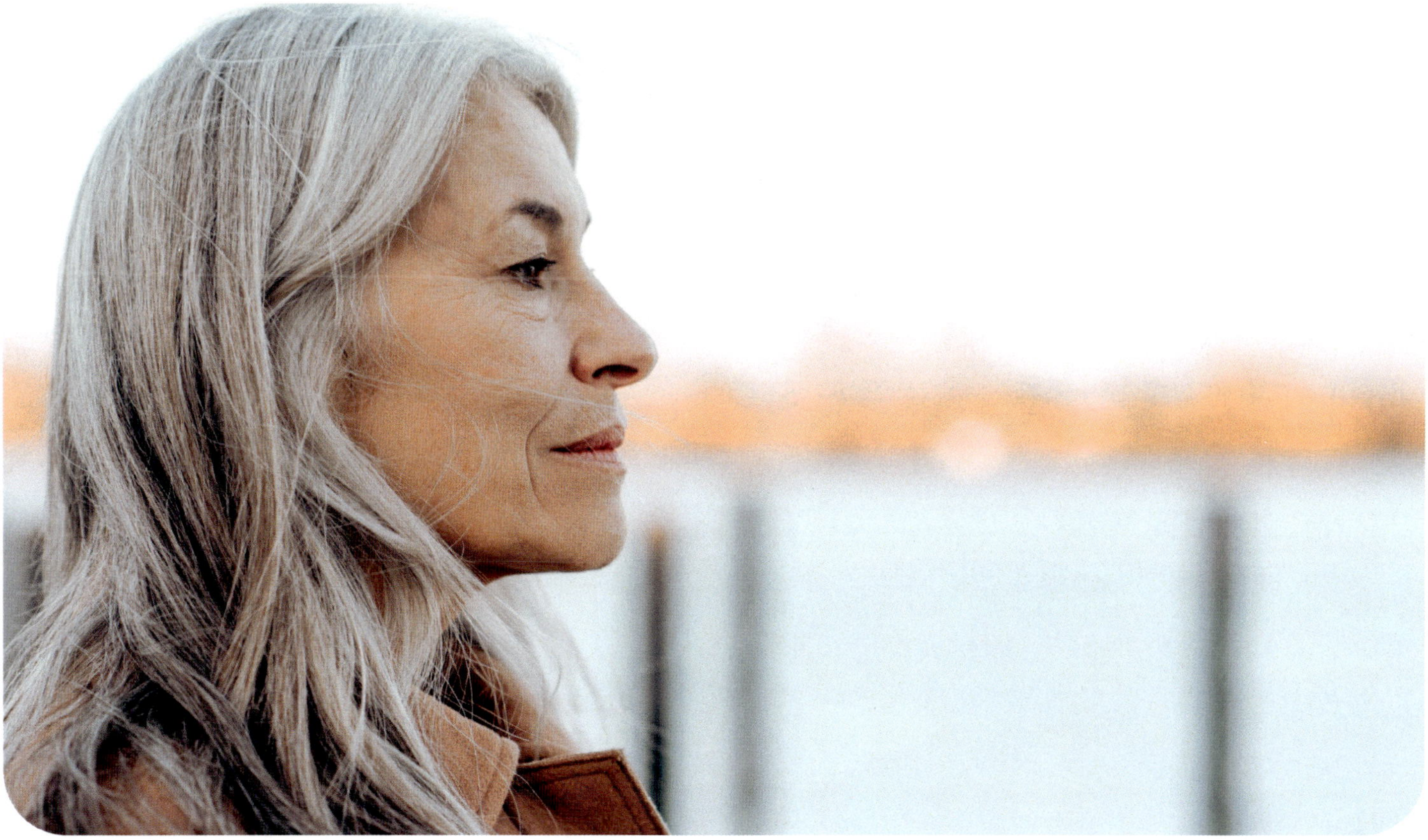

T-ALL includes a group of cancers that start in T-cell lymphocytes. It is less common than B-ALL and is Philadelphia chromosome-negative (Ph-). Treatment options include a clinical trial or systemic therapy.

Treatment

T-ALL is Ph-negative (Ph-). It does not have the Philadelphia chromosome. It is recommended that T-ALL be treated in a clinical trial when possible.

Induction

Induction chemotherapy might include daunorubicin, vincristine, prednisone, and pegaspargase.

All regimens include central nervous system (CNS) prophylaxis with systemic therapy and/or intrathecal (IT) therapy. Treatment response will be measured after completing induction. Tests will look for minimal residual disease (MRD).

Consolidation

Consolidation is a continuation of chemotherapy. Nelarabine might be added to a consolidation regimen. After consolidation, treatment response will be assessed.

Continuation therapy

The goal of extended maintenance or continuation therapy is to prevent cancer from returning (called a relapse) or spreading to the CNS or testicles, and to reduce the amount of MRD.

After continuation therapy, a stem cell transplant might be an option. However, an SCT depends upon donor availability and your health at the time of potential SCT.

Surveillance

After a complete response or a stem cell transplant, your will be monitored for signs of recurrence or relapse. Relapse is the return of cancer.

Relapse

T-ALL often returns. Relapse can occur in the bone marrow called isolated medullary relapse, in the testicles or central nervous system called isolated extramedullary relapse, or a combination of both. Isolated extramedullary relapse requires systemic therapy to prevent relapse in bone marrow.

Relapse treatment options:

- Clinical trial
- Systemic therapy

Treatments will likely include a combination of drugs. Relapse can happen multiple times. With each relapse the goal of treatment is a complete response or an MRD-negative result before an SCT.

Refractory

When leukemia remains and does not respond to treatment, it is called refractory or resistant. The cancer may be resistant at the start of treatment or it may become resistant during treatment. Refractory disease is very serious. It is important to ask about prognosis.

Refractory treatment options:

- Clinical trial
- Systemic therapy

The goal is to achieve an MRD-negative result before an SCT. However, in some cases an SCT might be considered in those who are MRD+.

Systemic therapy options for relapsed or refractory Ph- T-ALL can be found in Guide 9.

A clinical trial is recommended for anyone with T-ALL.

Guide 9
Systemic therapy options: Relapsed or refractory T-ALL

Preferred	• Nelarabine • Nelarabine with etoposide and cyclophosphamide
Other	• Bortezomib with chemotherapy (for AYA patients) • Daratumumab • High-dose cytarabine (HiDAC) • Mitoxantrone, etoposide, and cytarabine • Venetoclax with chemotherapy • Regimens for relapsed/refractory Ph- B-ALL may be appropriate

Review

- T-ALL includes a group of cancers that start in T-cell lymphocytes. T-ALL does not have the Philadelphia chromosome (Ph-).
- It is recommended that T-ALL be treated in a clinical trial when possible. Systemic therapy is also a treatment option. All regimens include central nervous system (CNS) prophylaxis with systemic therapy and/or intrathecal (IT) therapy.
- The goal of treatment is a complete response (CR).
- After a CR or a stem cell transplant (SCT), you will be monitored for signs of recurrence or relapse.
- When cancer returns or relapses, the goal of treatment is to have another CR. After a CR, an SCT might follow. An SCT depends upon donor availability and your health at the time of potential SCT.
- Cancer may be resistant at the start of treatment or it may become resistant during treatment. This is called refractory.

A stem cell transplant (SCT) depends upon donor availability and your health at the time of potential SCT.

8 Making treatment decisions

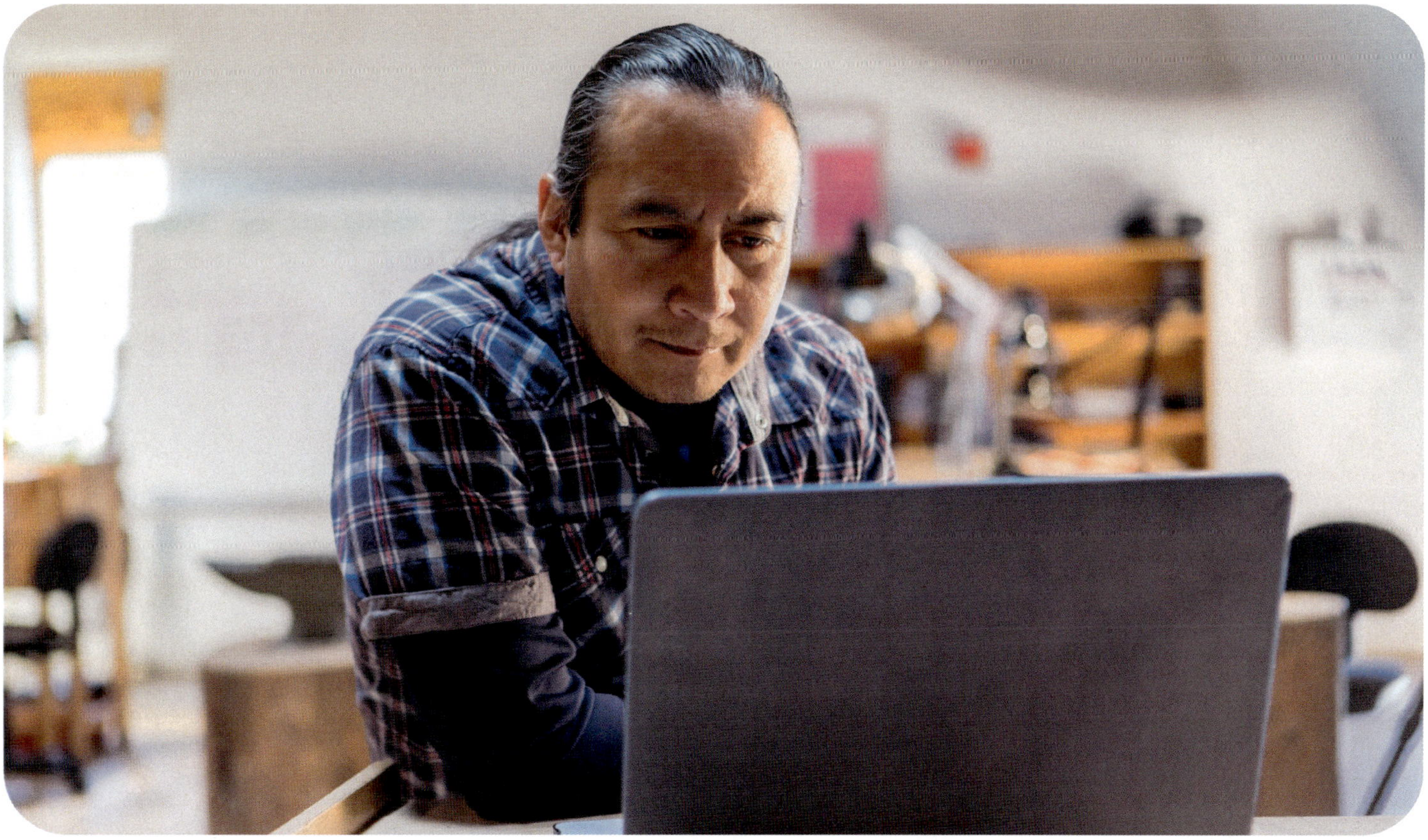

It's important to be comfortable with the cancer treatment you choose. This choice starts with having an open and honest conversation with your doctor.

It's your choice

In shared decision-making, you and your doctors share information, discuss the options, and agree on a treatment plan. It starts with an open and honest conversation between you and your doctor.

Treatment decisions are very personal. What is important to you may not be important to someone else.

Some things that may play a role in your decision-making:

- What you want and how that might differ from what others want
- Your religious and spiritual beliefs
- Your feelings about certain treatments like surgery or chemotherapy
- Your feelings about pain or side effects such as nausea and vomiting
- Cost of treatment, travel to treatment centers, and time away from school or work
- Quality of life and length of life
- How active you are and the activities that are important to you

Think about what you want from treatment. Discuss openly the risks and benefits of specific treatments and procedures. Weigh options and share concerns with your doctor. If you take the time to build a relationship with your doctor, it will help you feel supported when considering options and making treatment decisions.

Second opinion

It is normal to want to start treatment as soon as possible. While cancer can't be ignored, there is time to have another doctor review your test results and suggest a treatment plan. This is called getting a second opinion, and it's a normal part of cancer care. Even doctors get second opinions!

Things you can do to prepare:

- Check with your insurance company about its rules on second opinions. There may be out-of-pocket costs to see doctors who are not part of your insurance plan.
- Make plans to have copies of all your records sent to the doctor you will see for your second opinion.

Support groups

Many people diagnosed with cancer find support groups to be helpful. Support groups often include people at different stages of treatment. Some people may be newly diagnosed, while others may be finished with treatment. If your hospital or community doesn't have support groups for people with cancer, check out the websites listed in this book.

Questions to ask your doctors

Possible questions to ask your doctors are listed on the following pages. Feel free to use these questions or come up with your own. Be clear about your goals for treatment and find out what to expect from treatment.

Questions to ask about diagnosis and testing

1. What type of ALL do I have? What does this mean in terms of prognosis and treatment options?
2. Should I consider treatment at a pediatric center?
3. What tests are needed? What other tests do you recommend?
4. How soon will I know the results and who will explain them to me?
5. Where will the tests take place? How long will the tests take?
6. Is there a cancer center or hospital nearby that specializes in this type of cancer?
7. What will you do to make me comfortable during testing?
8. How do I prepare for testing? How will the test be done? What can I expect?
9. Would you give me a copy of the pathology report and other test results?
10. Who will talk with me about the next steps? When?
11. Will treatment start before the test results are in?
12. How many bone marrow tests are needed? When are they done?

Questions to ask about options

1. What will happen if I do nothing?
2. How do age, white blood cell (WBC) count, health, and other factors affect the options?
3. How will treatment affect my fertility? Should I see a fertility specialist before starting treatment?
4. Am I a candidate for a blood stem cell transplant?
5. Am I candidate for a clinical trial?
6. Which option is proven to work best for my ALL subtype, age, and other risk factors?
7. Does any option offer a cure or long-term cancer control? Are the chances any better for one option than another? Less time-consuming? Less expensive?
8. How do you know if treatment is working? How will I know if treatment is working?
9. What are my options if the treatment stops working?
10. Are there any life-threatening side effects of this treatment? How will these be monitored?
11. What should I expect from this treatment? How long will treatment last?
12. Can I stop treatment at any time? What will happen? How will I know when to stop blood transfusions or antibiotics?

Questions to ask about treatment

1. What are the treatment choices? What are the benefits and risks?
2. Which treatment do you recommend and why?
3. How long do I have to decide?
4. Will I have to go to the hospital or elsewhere for treatment? How often? How long is each visit? Will I have to stay overnight in the hospital or make travel plans?
5. Do I have a choice of when to begin treatment? Can I choose the days and times of treatment?
6. How much will the treatment hurt? What will you do to make me comfortable?
7. How much will this treatment cost? What does my insurance cover? Are there any programs to help pay for treatment?
8. What kind of treatment will I do at home? What can I do to prepare our home to ensure my safety or the safety of other family members in the household?
9. What can I do to prevent or relieve side effects? What will you do?
10. Which treatment will give me the best quality of life? Which treatment will extend life? By how long?
11. Will I miss school or work?
12. What in particular should be avoided or taken with caution while receiving treatment?

Questions to ask your doctors about their experience

1. What is your experience treating this type ALL?
2. What is the experience of those on your team?
3. Do you only treat adult ALL? What else do you treat?
4. I would like to get a second opinion. Is there someone you recommend?
5. I would like another pathologist or hematopathologist to review the blood samples. Is there someone you recommend?
6. How many patients like me (of the same age, gender, race) have you treated?
7. Will you be consulting with ALL experts to discuss my care? Whom will you consult?
8. How many procedures like the one you're suggesting have you done?
9. Is this treatment a major part of your practice?
10. How many of your patients have had complications? What were the complications?

Questions to ask about clinical trials

1. What clinical trials are available? Are we eligible for any of them? Why or why not?
2. What are the treatments used in the clinical trial?
3. What does the treatment do?
4. Has the treatment been used before? Has it been used for other types of cancer?
5. What are the risks and benefits of this treatment?
6. What side effects should I expect? How will the side effects be controlled?
7. How long will I be on the clinical trial?
8. Will I be able to have other treatment if this doesn't work?
9. How will you know the treatment is working?
10. Will the clinical trial cost me anything? If so, how much?

Questions to ask about stem cell transplants

1. How do you find a donor?
2. How long will I have to wait for a stem cell transplant (SCT)?
3. What do we need to do to prepare?
4. What will you do to prepare?
5. What are the risks to myself and/or the donor?
6. How will the transplant affect my prognosis?
7. How will a transplant affect the quality and length of my life?
8. What should I expect?
9. How long should I expect to be in the hospital?
10. How will I feel before, during, and after the transplant?
11. How many SCTs has this center done for those with this type of ALL?
12. Will I have more than one SCT?
13. What side effects may occur after an SCT?
14. Is radiation treatment included with an SCT?

Questions to ask about side effects

1. What are the side effects of treatment?
2. How long will these side effects last? Do any side effects lessen or worsen in severity over time?
3. What side effects should I watch for? What side effects are expected and which are life-threatening?
4. When should I call the doctor? Can I text?
5. What medicines can I take to prevent or relieve side effects?
6. What can I do to help with pain and other side effects?
7. Will you stop treatment or change treatment if there are side effects? What do you look for?
8. What can I do to lessen or prevent side effects? What will you do?
9. What side effects are life-long and irreversible even after completing treatment?
10. What medicines may worsen side effects of treatment?

Questions to ask about survivorship and late effects

1. What happens after treatment?
2. What are the chances ALL will return or that I will develop another type of cancer?
3. Whom do we see for follow-up care? How often?
4. Should I see a dentist? An eye doctor?
5. What tests will I have to monitor their health?
6. What late effects are caused by this treatment? How will these be screened? What should look for?
7. What should I do if I have trouble with work or school? Or difficulty focusing?
8. I am looking for a survivor support group. What support groups or other resources can you recommend?

Resources

American Association for Clinical Chemistry
labtestsonline.org

American Cancer Society
cancer.org/cancer/leukemia-in-children

American Society of Hematology
hematology.org/education/patients

Be The Match®
bethematch.org

Blood & Marrow Transplant Information Network
bmtinfonet.org

Cancer*Care*
cancercare.org

Chemocare
chemocare.com

MedlinePlus
medlineplus.gov

National Bone Marrow Transplant Link
nbmtlink.org

National Cancer Institute
cancer.gov/types/leukemia

cancer.gov/publications/patient-education/children-with-cancer.pdf

National Coalition for Cancer Survivorship
canceradvocacy.org/toolbox/

National Hospice and Palliative Care Organization
nhpco.org/patients-and-caregivers

OncoLink
oncolink.org

Radiological Society of North America
radiologyinfo.org

Stupid Cancer
stupidcancer.org

The Leukemia & Lymphoma Society
lls.org/leukemia/acute-lymphoblastic-leukemia/childhood-all

U.S. Department of Health & Human Services
bloodstemcell.hrsa.gov

Words to know

absolute neutrophil count (ANC)
An estimate of the body's ability to fight infections, especially bacterial infections.

adolescent and young adult (AYA)
People who are 15 to 39 years of age at the time of initial cancer diagnosis.

acute lymphoblastic leukemia (ALL)
A fast-growing cancer that causes too many immature white blood cells called lymphoblasts to be made.

antibody
A protein made by a plasma cell (a type of white blood cell).

autologous
Stem cells come from you.

allogeneic
Donor that may or may not be related to you.

B cell
A type of lymphocyte.

BCR-ABL1 protein
An abnormal protein that is made by the *BCR-ABL1* fusion gene and causes too many abnormal white blood cells to be made.

biopsy
A procedure that removes tissue samples.

blast
An immature blood cell. Also called lymphoblast.

blood stem cell
An immature blood-forming cell from which all other types of blood cells are made. Also called hematopoietic stem cell.

blood stem cell transplant (SCT)
A treatment that replaces damaged or diseased cells in the bone marrow with healthy blood-forming cells.

bone marrow
The soft, sponge-like tissue in the center of most bones where blood cells are made.

bone marrow aspirate
The removal of a small amount of liquid bone marrow to test for disease.

bone marrow biopsy
The removal of a small amount of solid bone and bone marrow to test for disease.

chemotherapy
Drugs that kill fast-growing cells, including cancer cells and normal cells.

chromosomes
Long strands that contain bundles of coded instructions in cells for making and controlling cells.

clinical trial
A study of how safe and helpful tests and treatments are for people.

computed tomography (CT)
A test that uses x-rays from many angles to make a picture of the insides of the body.

consolidation
The second stage of treatment.

contrast
A substance put into your body to make clearer pictures during imaging tests.

cytogenetics
The study of chromosomes.

deoxyribonucleic acid (DNA)
Long strands of genetic information found inside cells.

donor
A person who gives their organs, tissues, or cells to another person.

extramedullary
Outside the bone marrow.

gene
Coded instructions in cells for making new cells and controlling how cells behave.

hematopoietic stem cell transplant (HSCT)
A treatment that replaces damaged or diseased cells in the bone marrow with healthy blood-forming cells. Also called stem cell transplant (SCT).

hematopathologist
A doctor who specializes in blood diseases by looking at cells under a microscope.

hematologist
A doctor who's an expert in diseases of the blood.

hereditary
Passed down from parent to child through coded information in cells (genes).

hyperdiploidy
Leukemia cells with 51 to 67 chromosomes.

hypodiploidy
Leukemia cells with fewer than 44 chromosomes.

human leukocyte antigen (HLA)
Special proteins on the surface of cells that help the body to tell its own cells apart from foreign cells.

immune system
The body's natural defense against infection and disease.

immunotherapy
A treatment with drugs that help the body find and destroy cancer cells.

induction
The first stage of treatment.

infection
An illness caused by germs.

infusion
A method for delivering chemotherapy into the vein in a controlled manner.

intravenous (IV)
A method of giving drugs by a needle or tube inserted into a vein.

interventional radiologist
A doctor who is an expert in imaging tests and using image-guided tools to perform minimally invasive techniques to diagnose or treat disease.

leukapheresis
A procedure that separates leukocytes from the blood.

leukemia
A disease in which there are too many white blood cells.

liver function test (LFT)
A lab test that measures chemicals made or processed by the liver.

lymph node
A small, bean-shaped, disease-fighting structure.

lymphoblast
An immature lymphocyte. Also called blast.

lymphocyte
A type of white blood cell that is part of the immune system.

lymphoid
Referring to a type of white blood cell called a lymphocyte.

magnetic resonance imaging (MRI)
A test that uses radio waves and powerful magnets to make pictures of the insides of the body.

medical oncologist
A doctor who is an expert in cancer drugs.

medullary
In the bone marrow.

minimal residual disease (MRD)
Cancer that remains after treatment.

mutation
An abnormal change.

myeloid
Referring to a type of white blood cell called a granulocyte.

myelosuppression
A condition in which bone marrow activity is decreased, resulting in fewer red blood cells, white blood cells, and platelets.

natural killer (NK) cell
A type of lymphocyte.

oncologist
A doctor who is an expert in the treatment of cancer.

palliative care
Health care that includes symptom relief but not cancer treatment. Also sometimes called supportive care.

pathologist
A doctor who is an expert in testing cells and tissue to find disease.

pediatric
People who are 18 years of age or under at the time of initial diagnosis.

peripheral blood
Blood that circulates throughout the body.

Philadelphia chromosome (Ph)
An abnormal, short chromosome 22 that is formed when parts of chromosomes 9 and 22 switch with each other. The result is the *BCR-ABL1* fused gene.

physical exam
A study of the body by a health expert for signs of disease.

platelet
A type of blood cell that helps control bleeding. Also called thrombocyte.

polymerase chain reaction (PCR)
A lab process in which copies of a piece of DNA are made.

positron emission tomography (PET)
A test that uses radioactive material to see the shape and function of body parts.

predisposition syndrome
Certain genetic changes, or mutations, can increase a person's chances of developing cancer.

prognosis
The likely course and outcome of a disease.

progression
The growth or spread of cancer after being tested or treated.

radiation therapy (RT)
A treatment that uses high-energy rays.

radiologist
A doctor who is an expert in imaging tests.

recurrence
The return of cancer after a cancer-free period.

red blood cell (RBC)
A type of blood cell that carries oxygen from the lungs to the rest of the body. Also called an erythrocyte.

refractory
A cancer that does not improve with treatment.

relapse
The return or worsening of cancer after a period of improvement.

regimen
A treatment plan that includes specific information about drug dose, when medicine is taken, and how long treatment will last.

remission
There are minor or no signs of a disease.

resistance
When cancer does not respond to a drug treatment.

scrotal ultrasound
Uses sound waves to make images of the scrotum. The scrotum is the pouch of skin at the base of the penis that contains the testicles.

side effect
An unhealthy or unpleasant physical or emotional response to treatment.

stem cell transplant (SCT)
A cancer treatment that destroys bone marrow and the replaces it by adding healthy blood stem cells. Also called hematopoietic stem cell transplant (HSCT) or bone marrow transplant (BMT).

steroid
A drug used to reduce redness, swelling, and pain, but also to kill cancer cells.

subtype
A smaller group within a type of cancer that is based on certain cell features.

supportive care
Health care that includes symptom relief but not cancer treatment. Also called palliative care or best supportive care.

surveillance
Testing that is done after treatment ends to check for the return of cancer.

systemic therapy
Treatment that works throughout the body.

T cell
A type of lymphocyte.

targeted therapy
A drug treatment that targets and attacks specific cancer cells.

translocation
When pieces of two chromosomes (long strands of coded instructions for controlling cells) break off and switch with each other.

tumor lysis syndrome (TLS)
A condition caused when waste released by dead cells is not quickly cleared out of the body.

tumor marker
A substance found in body tissue or fluid that may be a sign of cancer.

white blood cell (WBC)
A type of blood cell that helps fight infections in the body. Also called a leukocyte.

NCCN Contributors

This patient guide is based on the NCCN Clinical Practice Guidelines in Oncology (NCCN Guidelines®) for Acute Lymphoblastic Leukemia. It was adapted, reviewed, and published with help from the following people:

Dorothy A. Shead, MS
Senior Director, Patient Information Operations

Rachael Clarke
Senior Medical Copyeditor

Tanya Fischer, MEd, MSLIS
Medical Writer

Laura J. Hanisch, PsyD
Medical Writer/Patient Information Specialist

Stephanie Helbling, MPH, CHES®
Medical Writer

Susan Kidney
Graphic Design Specialist

John Murphy
Medical Writer

Erin Vidic, MA
Medical Writer

Kim Williams
Creative Services Manager

The NCCN Guidelines® for Acute Lymphoblastic Leukemia Version 1.2021 were developed by the following NCCN Panel Members:

Patrick A. Brown, MD/Chair
The Sidney Kimmel Comprehensive Cancer Center at Johns Hopkins

Bijal Shah, MD/Vice-Chair
Moffitt Cancer Center

*Anjali Advani, MD
Case Comprehensive Cancer Center/ University Hospitals Seidman Cancer Center and Cleveland Clinic Taussig Cancer Institute

Patricia Aoun, MD, MPH
City of Hope National Medical Center

Bhavana Bhatnagar, DO
The Ohio State University Comprehensive Cancer Center - James Cancer Hospital and Solove Research Institute

*Michael W. Boyer, MD
Huntsman Cancer Institute at the University of Utah

Patrick W. Burke, MD
University of Michigan Rogel Cancer Center

Ryan D. Cassaday, MD
Fred Hutchinson Cancer Research Center/ Seattle Cancer Care Alliance

Daniel J. DeAngelo, MD, PhD
Dana-Farber/Brigham and Women's Cancer Center

*Shira Dinner, MD
Robert H. Lurie Comprehensive Cancer Center of Northwestern University

Amir T. Fathi, MD
Massachusetts General Hospital Cancer Center

Jordan Gauthier, MD, MSc
Fred Hutchinson Cancer Research Center/ Seattle Cancer Care Alliance

Nitin Jain, MD
The University of Texas MD Anderson Cancer Center

Suzanne Kirby, MD
Duke Cancer Institute

Michaela Liedtke, MD
Stanford Cancer Institute

Mark Litzow, MD
Mayo Clinic Cancer Center

Aaron Logan, MD, PhD
UCSF Helen Diller Family Comprehensive Cancer Center

*Selina Luger, MD
Abramson Cancer Center at the University of Pennsylvania

Lori J Maness, MD
Fred & Pamela Buffett Cancer Center

Stephanie Massaro, MD, MPH
Yale Cancer Center/Smilow Cancer Hospital

Ryan J. Mattison, MD
University of Wisconsin Carbone Cancer Center

William May, MD
UCLA Jonsson Comprehensive Cancer Center

Olalekan Oluwole, MD
Vanderbilt-Ingram Cancer Center

Jae Park, MD
Memorial Sloan Kettering Cancer Center

Amanda Przespolewski, DO
Roswell Park Comprehensive Cancer Center

Sravanti Rangaraju, MD
O'Neal Comprehensive Cancer Center at UAB

Jeffrey E. Rubnitz, MD, PhD
St. Jude Children's Research Hospital/ The University of Tennessee Health Science Center

Geoffrey L. Uy, MD
Siteman Cancer Center at Barnes-Jewish Hospital and Washington University School of Medicine

Madhuri Vusirikala, MD
UT Southwestern Simmons Comprehensive Cancer Center

Matthew Wieduwilt, MD, PhD
UC San Diego Moores Cancer Center

NCCN Staff

Beth Lynn RN, BS, CMSRN
Guidelines Layout Specialist

Ndiya Ogba, PhD
Oncology Scientist/Senior Medical Writer

* Reviewed this patient guide.
For disclosures, visit NCCN.org/about/disclosure.aspx.

NCCN Cancer Centers

Abramson Cancer Center
at the University of Pennsylvania
Philadelphia, Pennsylvania
800.789.7366 • pennmedicine.org/cancer

Fred & Pamela Buffett Cancer Center
Omaha, Nebraska
402.559.5600 • unmc.edu/cancercenter

Case Comprehensive Cancer Center/
University Hospitals Seidman Cancer
Center and Cleveland Clinic Taussig
Cancer Institute
Cleveland, Ohio
800.641.2422 • UH Seidman Cancer Center
uhhospitals.org/services/cancer-services
866.223.8100 • CC Taussig Cancer Institute
my.clevelandclinic.org/departments/cancer
216.844.8797 • Case CCC
case.edu/cancer

City of Hope National Medical Center
Los Angeles, California
800.826.4673 • cityofhope.org

Dana-Farber/Brigham and
Women's Cancer Center
Boston, Massachusetts
617.732.5500
youhaveus.org

Massachusetts General Hospital
Cancer Center
617.726.5130
massgeneral.org/cancer-center

Duke Cancer Institute
Durham, North Carolina
888.275.3853 • dukecancerinstitute.org

Fox Chase Cancer Center
Philadelphia, Pennsylvania
888.369.2427 • foxchase.org

Huntsman Cancer Institute
at the University of Utah
Salt Lake City, Utah
800.824.2073
huntsmancancer.org

Fred Hutchinson Cancer
Research Center/Seattle
Cancer Care Alliance
Seattle, Washington
206.606.7222 • seattlecca.org
206.667.5000 • fredhutch.org

The Sidney Kimmel Comprehensive
Cancer Center at Johns Hopkins
Baltimore, Maryland
410.955.8964
hopkinskimmelcancercenter.org

Robert H. Lurie Comprehensive
Cancer Center of Northwestern
University
Chicago, Illinois
866.587.4322 • cancer.northwestern.edu

Mayo Clinic Cancer Center
Phoenix/Scottsdale, Arizona
Jacksonville, Florida
Rochester, Minnesota
480.301.8000 • Arizona
904.953.0853 • Florida
507.538.3270 • Minnesota
mayoclinic.org/cancercenter

Memorial Sloan Kettering
Cancer Center
New York, New York
800.525.2225 • mskcc.org

Moffitt Cancer Center
Tampa, Florida
888.663.3488 • moffitt.org

The Ohio State University
Comprehensive Cancer Center -
James Cancer Hospital and
Solove Research Institute
Columbus, Ohio
800.293.5066 • cancer.osu.edu

O'Neal Comprehensive
Cancer Center at UAB
Birmingham, Alabama
800.822.0933 • uab.edu/onealcancercenter

Roswell Park Comprehensive
Cancer Center
Buffalo, New York
877.275.7724 • roswellpark.org

Siteman Cancer Center at Barnes-
Jewish Hospital and Washington
University School of Medicine
St. Louis, Missouri
800.600.3606 • siteman.wustl.edu

St. Jude Children's Research Hospital
The University of Tennessee
Health Science Center
Memphis, Tennessee
866.278.5833 • stjude.org
901.448.5500 • uthsc.edu

Stanford Cancer Institute
Stanford, California
877.668.7535 • cancer.stanford.edu

UC Davis
Comprehensive Cancer Center
Sacramento, California
916.734.5959 | 800.770.9261
health.ucdavis.edu/cancer

UC San Diego Moores Cancer Center
La Jolla, California
858.822.6100• cancer.ucsd.edu

UCLA Jonsson
Comprehensive Cancer Center
Los Angeles, California
310.825.5268 • cancer.ucla.edu

UCSF Helen Diller Family
Comprehensive Cancer Center
San Francisco, California
800.689.8273 • cancer.ucsf.edu

University of Colorado Cancer Center
Aurora, Colorado
720.848.0300 • coloradocancercenter.org

University of Michigan
Rogel Cancer Center
Ann Arbor, Michigan
800.865.1125 • rogelcancercenter.org

The University of Texas
MD Anderson Cancer Center
Houston, Texas
844.269.5922 • mdanderson.org

University of Wisconsin
Carbone Cancer Center
Madison, Wisconsin
608.265.1700 • uwhealth.org/cancer

UT Southwestern Simmons
Comprehensive Cancer Center
Dallas, Texas
214.648.3111 • utsouthwestern.edu/simmons

Vanderbilt-Ingram Cancer Center
Nashville, Tennessee
877.936.8422 • vicc.org

Yale Cancer Center/
Smilow Cancer Hospital
New Haven, Connecticut
855.4.SMILOW • yalecancercenter.org

Notes

Index

Made in the USA
Coppell, TX
05 November 2026

11302976R00052